Visit our website

to find out about other books from W. B. Saunders
and our sister companies in Harcourt Health Sciences

Register free at
www.harcourt-international.com

and you will get

- the latest information on new books, journals and electronic products in your chosen subject areas

- the choice of e-mail or post alerts or both, when there are any new books in your chosen areas

- news of special offers and promotions

- information about products from all Harcourt Health Sciences' companies including Baillière Tindall, Churchill Livingstone, Mosby and W. B. Saunders

You will also find an easily searchable catalogue, online ordering, information on our extensive list of journals...and much more!

Visit the Harcourt Health Sciences' website today!

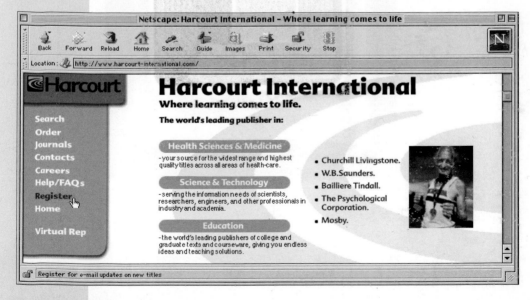

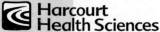

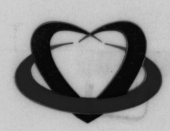

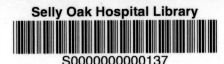
Imaging for Junior Doctors

Commissioning Editor: Michael J. Houston
Development Editor: Sheila Black
Project Manager: Cheryl Brant
Production Controller: Helen Sofio
Designer: Ian Dick

Imaging for Junior Doctors
A Survival Guide

Peter Kember MB ChB MRCP (UK) FRCR
Consultant Radiologist, Department of Radiology, Torbay Hospital,
Torquay, UK

W. B. SAUNDERS COMPANY

London Edinburgh New York Philadelphia St Louis Sydney Toronto 2000

WB SAUNDERS
An imprint of Harcourt Publishers Limited

© Harcourt Publishers Limited 2000

 is a registered trademark of Harcourt Publishers Limited

The right of Peter Kember to be identified as the author of this work has been asserted by him in accordance with the Copyright, Designs and Patents Act 1988.

First published 2000

ISBN 0 7020 2498 8

British Library Cataloguing in Publication Data
A catalogue record for this book is available from the British Library

Library of Congress Cataloging in Publication Data
A catalog record for this book is available from the Library of Congress

Note
Medical knowledge is constantly changing. As new information becomes available, changes in treatment, procedures, equipment and the use of drugs become necessary. The editors/authors/contributors and the publishers have, as far as it is possible, taken care to ensure that the information given in this text is accurate and up to date. However, readers are strongly advised to confirm that the information, especially with regard to drug usage, complies with the latest legislation and standards of practice.

The
publisher's
policy is to use
**paper manufactured
from sustainable forests**

Printed in China
SWTC/01

Contents

Dedication

For my parents, and for Kathy, William and Lucy.

Acknowledgements

I owe thanks to a number of people; Richard Nakielny and Mike Collins in Sheffield and Maria Khan at WB Saunders provided encouragement and sound advice from the outset. Michael Houston, at Harcourt Publishers, has supported the project enthusiastically through to completion. My colleagues John Isaacs, Richard Seymour, Richard Bolton, Richard Heafield, Lyn Morris and Sarah Horton have contributed greatly and helped with a number of the illustrations. I am also indebted to the many radiographers, clerical and darkroom staff at Torbay for their tireless help in finding and copying the films used in the book.

Introduction

Few junior doctors will get through their first day without requesting an X-ray of some variety, and many will have to make a decision on the patient's immediate management based on their interpretation of the film. And yet radiology is largely undertaught at medical schools, and the difficulty of plain film interpretation is often underestimated.

This book aims to answer two questions: (1) What test should I request? (2) What should I look for on the film?

Patients do not present with their diagnosis written on their foreheads, so it is much more relevant to know how to investigate a specific symptom and what to look for on the X-ray than to know the X-ray appearances of (for example) Wegener's granulomatosis. I have therefore adopted a symptom-based approach.

X-rays have been around for over a century now, and will undoubtedly continue to be widely used in this millennium for the foreseeable future. The development of CT, Ultrasound and MRI has added considerably to the radiologist's armoury, but the plain X-ray remains the first imaging test for the majority of patients. I make no apology therefore for devoting most of the book's content to plain X-rays. These, after all, are the films which junior doctors have to interpret, often in the early hours when most radiologists are tucked up in bed dreaming of MRI scans. The exception to this is the second chapter where CTs outnumber skull X-rays by 10:1 – and so they should. I have not included A&E type trauma much; for this I refer the reader to the excellent book by Raby, Berman and deLacey (*Accident and Emergency Radiology – A Survival Guide*, London: WB Saunders, 1995).

PK
2000

Abbreviations

AP	antero-posterior		LLL	left lower lobe
AV	arteriovenous		LP	lumbar puncture
AVM	arteriovenous malformation		LV	left ventricular
			LUL	left upper lobe
CABG	coronary artery bypass graft			
CBD	common bile duct		MDP	methylene diphosphate
CF	cystic fibrosis		MI	myocardial infarction
COPD	chronic obstructive pulmonary disease		MTP	metatarso-phalangeal (joint)
CSF	cerebral spinal fluid		NG	nasogastric
CVA	cerebrovascular accident			
CXR	chest X-ray		PA	postero-anterior
			PCA	posterior cerebral artery
D&C	dilatation & curettage		PE	pulmonary embolism
DIP	distal interphalangeal (joint)		PR	per rectum
DVT	deep vein thrombosis		PTC	percutaneous transhepatic cholangiogram
ERCP	endoscopic retrograde cholangio-pancreatogram		PV	per vaginal
ET	endotracheal		RBC	red blood cell
			RIF	right iliac fossa
FBC	full blood count		RLL	right lower lobe
FESS	functional endoscopic sinus surgery		RML	right middle lobe
			RTA	road traffic accident
			RUL	right upper lobe
GI	gastrointestinal			
			SHO	senior house officer
IMA	interior mesenteric artery		SI	sacro-iliac (joint)
ITU	intensive therapy unit		SMA	superior mesenteric artery
IVC	interior vena cava		SVC	superior vena cava
IVU	intravenous urogram		SXR	skull X-ray

Imaging techniques

1

X-rays are produced when electrons hit a tungsten anode target in an evacuated tube. A focused beam of X-rays is directed through the patient and onto a cassette containing an intensifying screen and a film. The X-rays are attenuated (reduced in intensity) as they pass through the patient, the degree of attenuation depending on the density of the patient. The X-rays which emerge from the patient hit the intensifying screen and produce light, which exposes the film.

CT (computed tomography) uses multiple X-ray sources and detectors, the data from which is used to produce a computerized cross-sectional image of the body. These images show not only the bone but also the solid organs and soft tissues with high resolution. New generation 'spiral' scanners are very fast; the entire thorax can be scanned in a single breath-hold, and reformatting of the images in any plane or in 3-D can be performed.

The problem with X-rays is their malignant potential. Although the risk should not be overstated, there is no safe dose, and the higher the dose the greater the risk. CT, barium studies and angiography are all high-dose procedures; it is our responsibility to use these techniques wisely. An examination involving radiation should only be requested if the findings, negative or positive, will help in the patient's further management.

Ultrasound carries no radiation and no such risk. The solid organs within the abdomen and pelvis can be beautifully seen; doppler scanning has become the imaging method of choice for assessing the swollen calf, the carotid artery bifurcation and the lower limb in arterial disease both pre- and post-operatively. Ultrasound is quick and easy to perform, but only by someone who finds ultrasound quick and easy to perform. This takes training and considerable experience, which is not always appreciated by clinicians keen to 'have a go at it'. Ultrasound often augments CT rather than being inferior to it. This is not always appreciated by clinicians either because, unlike the beautiful pictures from a CT, the hard-copy images from an ultrasound examination are difficult to interpret by anyone other than the person who did the scan. As well as being operator dependent, ultrasound is much more patient dependent than CT; hence the occasional report 'the scan was compromised by the patient's obesity…'.

MRI (magnetic resonance imaging) is the radiologist's exciting new toy for the new millennium, although it has been around for some 10 or 15 years now. Its availability has increased significantly over the last five years, such that most departments now have an on-site magnet or regular access to a mobile scanner (on the back of an articulated lorry). MRI uses no radiation and carries no known risk to date. The patient is placed in a very powerful magnet which aligns the protons in his or her body in the direction of the magnetic field. Brief radio-frequency pulses deflect the protons, and they are then allowed to return to alignment, the time taken to do so being determined by the make-up of the tissue. The difference in this 'relaxation time' between tissues is what the computerized image is based upon. MRI can produce images in any plane which have much greater contrast resolution than CT, although spatial resolution is inferior; i.e. differentiation between soft tissues of similar density is much better, but the images are 'grainier'. In practice this means that an MRI of the knee shows the ligaments, menisci and joint cartilage all in exquisite detail. MRI is now king for musculoskeletal and neurological imaging, and is increasingly making in-roads in other areas such as arteriography and cholangiography, which can be performed totally noninvasively. Having said that, it is unlikely that MRI will do away with the more conventional techniques in all areas. The main disadvantage of MRI is the comparatively long scanning time, requiring the patient to remain still for anything up to one hour in the cramped and noisy confines of the scanner. There are also specific contraindications to MRI; namely the presence of a permanent pacemaker, ferromagnetic aneurysm clip or intraocular metallic foreign body. A small but significant minority of patients also have problems with claustrophobia.

Radioisotope tests involve the injection of a material which has a radioactive isotope attached, most commonly technetium-99. The carrier material determines the site to which the isotope is delivered, e.g in a lung scan Tc-labelled microspheres are trapped in the pulmonary capillaries, in a bone scan Tc-labelled MDP is taken up by bone. The patient then lies on a gamma camera, producing an image determined by the distribution of the radioisotope. As with X-rays and CT, the radiation dose must always be considered when requesting these examinations.

The head

2

IMAGING TECHNIQUES

AP and lateral *skull X-rays* are usually performed with the patient lying supine. A *Towne's view* is also obtained in trauma cases to demonstrate the occipital bone.

A *CT head scan* (Fig. 2.1) is performed with the patient lying supine in the scanner. Slices 8–10 mm thick through the brain are usually obtained, with thinner (4–5 mm) slices through the posterior fossa. Scanning time is usually only a few minutes, but this still demands a patient who is able to lie still; a confused or fitting patient may therefore need sedating. Most scans are performed without IV contrast, which can mask acute haemorrhage. A contrast-enhanced scan may then be performed to assess enhancement of any mass lesions identified. The brain is visualized in considerable detail with the possible exception of the posterior fossa, the bony confines of which result in some image degradation. CT scanning remains the investigation of choice in head trauma, acute stroke and intracerebral

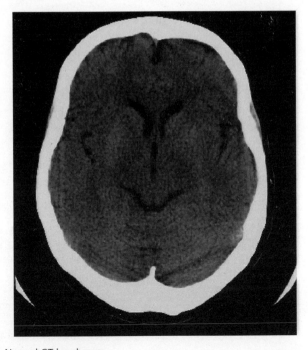

Fig. 2.1 Normal CT head scan.

haemorrhage. In other conditions MRI often complements rather than replaces CT.

An *MRI brain scan* (Fig. 2.2) is performed in a similar manner to CT, although patients are more prone to claustrophobia within the tighter confines of the scanner. A typical scan takes 5 min per sequence, with two to three sequences usually being performed; some patients require sedation. Modern nonferrous aneurysm clips are safe for scanning purposes, but older ferromagnetic clips are contraindicated due to the risk of clip motion. Intraocular foreign bodies (e.g. in sheet-metal workers) are also a contraindication. Contrast enhancement with gadolinium is used in a similar manner to CT scanning. MRI is much more sensitive than CT in detecting cerebral oedema, encephalitis, plaques of demyelination and acute infarcts (Fig. 2.3). In addition the ability to scan in any anatomical plane is often helpful in the assessment of mass lesions. *Magnetic resonance angiography* (MRA) (Fig. 2.4) employs specific sequences to image the intracranial blood vessels. Although it has not replaced the 'gold standard' of conventional angiography (yet), it does allow detailed visualization of cerebral vessels without the need for complex arterial catheterization.

Cerebral angiography allows the cerebral arteries to be visualized in exquisite detail. It can usually be performed using local anaesthesia

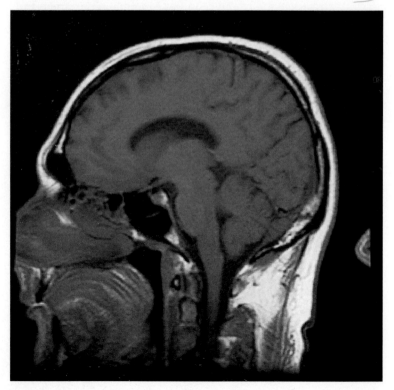

Fig. 2.2 Normal MRI brain scan. Midsagittal T1-weighted image.

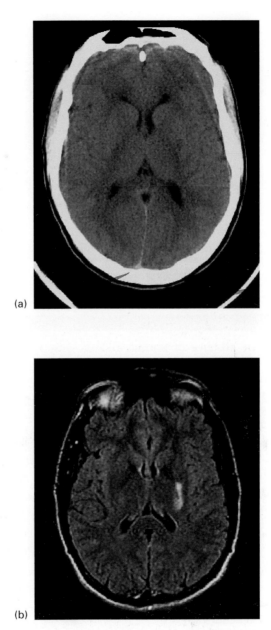

Fig. 2.3 Small infarct: CT (a) vs MRI (b). A very small acute infarct is only just discernable on CT, but is strikingly obvious on an MRI performed the following day.

only. A catheter inserted via the femoral artery is positioned with its tip in the carotid and vertebral arteries in turn. Rapid sequence exposures are taken during a hand injection of iodinated contrast. Exposures taken after a short time delay allow the venous circulation to be imaged. The main complication is stroke, but its incidence is less than 1%.

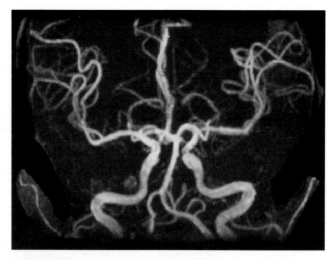

Fig. 2.4 Normal MRA of the cerebral circulation.

HEADACHE

In the absence of trauma a skull X-ray is not indicated. Although very occasionally it may point to an underlying abnormality (e.g. when there is shift of the calcified pineal gland away from the midline due to mass effect from a tumour) this is uncommon, and even then CT is still required.

Most patients with headache do not have a brain tumour. The decision to investigate depends primarily on the history and the presence of focal neurological signs or raised intracranial pressure. One exception to this rule is an acute onset severe headache suggestive of subarachnoid haemorrhage. CT scan is the investigation of choice.

Migraine

Unless there are atypical features in the history or on clinical examination, head scanning is *not* indicated. CT is normal except in the rare case of cerebral artery occlusion (usually PCA) complicating a severe attack.

Cranial arteritis

As with migraine, if the history and examination are typical there is no indication to perform a CT scan, which will show no abnormality.

Sinusitis

Although the paranasal sinuses may show mucosal thickening and fluid collections, both on CT and on skull X-rays, the correlation with symptoms is poor; these appearances are frequently encountered in asymptomatic individuals. When the diagnosis has been made clinically, CT is rarely indicated, i.e. when extension of infection into the adjacent cranial fossa is suspected. However, coronal CT scans of the paranasal sinuses are commonly performed in chronic cases prior to functional endoscopic sinus surgery (FESS).

Meningitis

Uncomplicated acute pyogenic meningitis is usually associated with a normal CT scan and is not in itself an indication to scan. Often in this situation CT is requested 'to exclude raised intracranial pressure prior to lumbar puncture', i.e. so not to cause coning. In practice if the fundi are normal and there are no clinical pointers to raised ICP, then CT is not routinely indicated; in any case a normal scan does not totally exclude raised ICP. Where the diagnosis is already known, the main indication for scanning is to look for the following complications:

■ Hydrocephalus: dilated ventricles due to obstructed CSF flow. The temporal horns are the first to enlarge.
■ Abscess collections: fluid collections in the subdural and parafalcine spaces.

Further imaging:

■ *Follow-up CT scans:* to assess progression of the aforementioned complications.

Encephalitis (Herpes simplex type 1)

Note that CT is usually *normal* in the first few days of this serious infection, even in the presence of severe neurological impairment. Subsequently:

■ Low density in temporal lobe: usually unilateral, may be bilateral (but asymmetric).
■ Associated mass effect: due to oedema.
■ Associated haemorrhage: in severe cases.

Further imaging:

■ *MRI* (Fig. 2.5) is the investigation of choice; it is much more sensitive than CT at detecting the oedema, which can be seen within 48–72 h.

Cerebral abscess (Fig. 2.6)

This is most commonly due to direct extension from sinusitis, middle ear infection or penetrating trauma. In IV drug abusers and suppurative lung disease they follow blood-borne spread. CT features:

■ Abscess mass lesion: if due to direct extension will be adjacent to

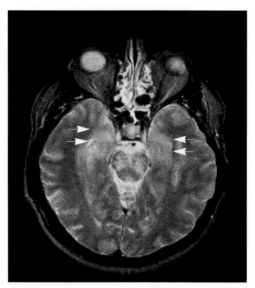

Fig. 2.5 Herpes simplex encephalitis. T2-weighted MRI showing bilateral high signal change in the medial aspects of the temporal lobes (arrows).

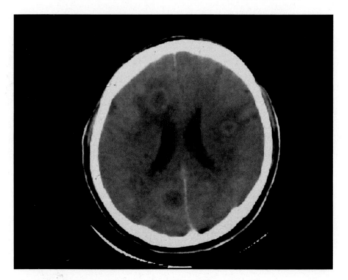

Fig. 2.6 Multiple cerebral abscesses, contrast-enhanced CT.

the underlying pathology. Blood-borne lesions may be multiple, and occur at the interface between grey and white matter particularly in the middle cerebral artery territory. As such they may closely resemble cerebral metastases.

■ Wall enhancement following IV contrast: this does not occur until a capsule has formed, after 1–2 weeks. Thereafter a very frequent finding, but does not correlate with infective activity.

■ Mass effect: displaces structures away from the abscess.

- Oedema: low density within the white matter.
- Gas: within the abscess itself is rare. When seen it has usually been introduced by surgery or is due to communication with an air sinus, rather than gas-forming organisms.

Further imaging:

- *Follow-up scans* to monitor response to therapy/surgery.

Subarachnoid haemorrhage (Fig. 2.7)

Most cases are due to spontaneous rupture of a berry aneurysm of the circle of Willis. Bleeding from AV malformations and trauma account for the remainder. CT findings:

- Blood in subarachnoid space: high density in the CSF spaces around the brainstem, in the Sylvian and interhemispheric fissures and sometimes within the ventricles. When localized can point to the site of the aneurysm, e.g. blood in the anterior interhemispheric fissure is usually from an

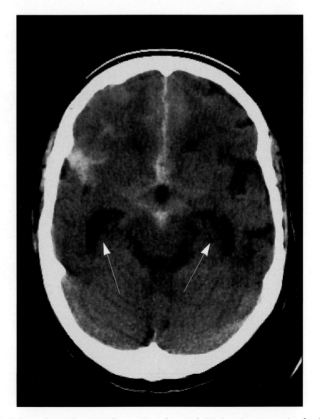

Fig. 2.7 Subarachnoid haemorrhage. Unenhanced CT showing extensive fresh blood (white) in the subarachnoid space. The temporal horns of the lateral ventricles are dilated due to secondary hydrocephalus (arrows).

anterior communicating or anterior cerebral artery aneurysm.

■ Hydrocephalus: due to obstruction to CSF flow. The temporal horns are the first to enlarge.

■ Normal scan: seen in approximately 5% of cases and more likely when there is a delay in scanning. An LP should be performed in these patients to completely exclude the diagnosis.

Further imaging:

■ *Cerebral angiography* to identify the aneurysm or AVM. This is usually performed within the first 48 h.

■ *MRA* as a noninvasive alternative to conventional angiography.

■ *Follow-up scans* as appropriate, depending on the clinical course.

Brain tumour

An account of all the different types of brain tumour is beyond the scope of this text. However, the three commonest account for over two-thirds of cases:

Gliomas (35%) (Fig. 2.8)

The commonest intracranial tumour, and astrocytomas are the commonest type. Very variable appearances due to very variable

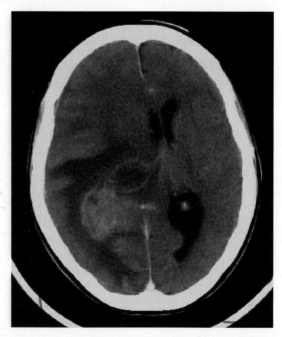

Fig. 2.8 Glioma, contrast-enhanced CT. A partly solid, partly cystic enhancing tumour with considerable oedema and mass effect. Note the displacement of the lateral ventricles.

malignancy. Relatively benign examples (Grade 1) tend to be well defined, are more commonly calcified and have little associated oedema. They show little or no contrast enhancement because the blood–brain barrier is intact. High-grade tumours (Grades 3 and 4, also called 'glioblastoma multiforme') are often multifocal, ill-defined and associated with considerable oedema. They show much more marked contrast enhancement and are more prone to spontaneous haemorrhage.

Meningiomas (15%) (Fig. 2.9)

The commonest benign intracranial tumour. They arise from the arachnoid covering of the dura mater. On CT they are well-defined high-density tumours which show marked contrast enhancement. Calcification occurs in up to 20% and may be dense enough to be visible on an SXR. The skull vault adjacent to the tumour may show a dense response termed hyperostosis which is also visible on a skull X-ray.

Metastases (20%) (Fig. 2.10)

Lung and breast carcinoma are the commonest primaries. A solitary cerebral metastasis occurs in up to 50% of cases; when there is no known primary malignancy this may make diagnosis difficult. CT appearances are variable, but they occur most commonly at the grey/white matter interface, show significant ring contrast enhancement and oedema, and are virtually never calcified.

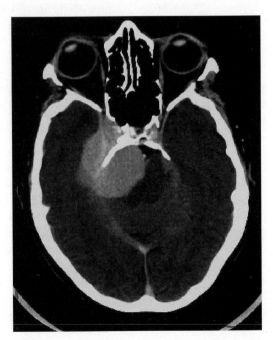

Fig. 2.9 Meningioma, contrast-enhanced CT. Note the well-defined uniformly enhancing appearance.

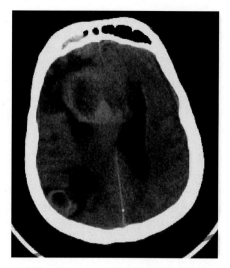

Fig. 2.10 Multiple cerebral metastases, unenhanced CT. These metastases are unusually dense (i.e. white on CT) which is typical of metastases from malignant melanoma.

Further imaging:

■ *MRI* (Fig. 2.11): although CT will demonstrate most brain tumours very clearly MRI is often valuable, particularly prior to surgery. The ability to perform coronal and sagittal images allows a clear demonstration of the anatomy of the lesion, and complications such as venous sinus invasion and spread within the CSF spaces is more readily seen. MRI is also more sensitive, demonstrating small tumours before they are evident on CT.
■ *Angiography* may be required prior to surgery.
■ *CXR* is mandatory to exclude a primary lung tumour.
■ *Follow-up scans*, e.g. to look for post-operative recurrence.

Pituitary tumours

Hormonally active tumours usually present early due to their endocrine effects. These tumours are usually < 1 cm, and are termed microadenomas. Hormonally inactive pituitary tumours do not present until large enough to produce pressure effects, either on the pituitary gland itself, causing hypopituitarism, or on the optic chiasm, causing visual field defects. Both micro- and macroadenomas are best imaged by MRI (Figs 2.12 and 2.13). CT is markedly inferior, and should only be reserved for patients with a contraindication to MRI.

TIAS AND STROKE

The symptoms and signs are dependent on the cerebral territory involved, but a vascular event is suggested when the onset is acute.

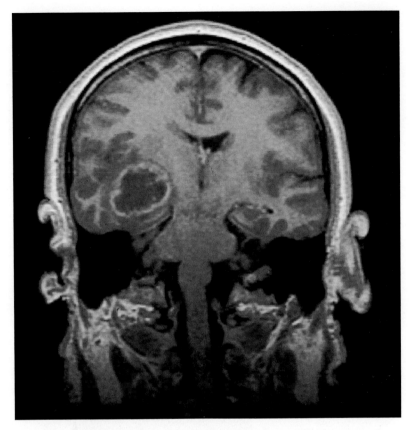

Fig. 2.11 Intracerebral tumour. Coronal MRI showing a ring enhancing tumour in the right temporal lobe. Note the compression of the lateral ventricle.

Imaging is not mandatory; when the clinical diagnosis is clear and anticoagulation is not being considered, then management will not be altered by the knowledge that the stroke is an infarct or a haemorrhage. Where definitive diagnosis is needed an unenhanced CT scan is the investigation of choice.

TIA

By definition a transient event which is not associated with any CT abnormality. However, there may be evidence of previous completed infarcts at other sites.

Further imaging:

■ *CXR ± echocardiography* are frequently requested to look for cardiovascular disease as a possible source of emboli. They are almost invariably normal.
■ *Carotid artery Doppler ultrasound* to look for stenosis and atheromatous plaque at the common carotid bifurcation.

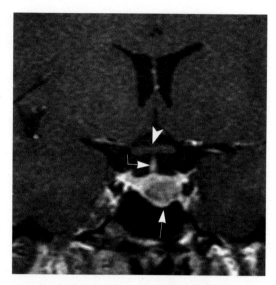

Fig. 2.12 Pituitary microadenoma. Contrast-enhanced coronal TI scan showing an 8 mm diameter tumour in the left side of the gland (arrow). Note that it is not displacing the pituitary stalk (curved arrow) or optic chiasm (arrowhead).

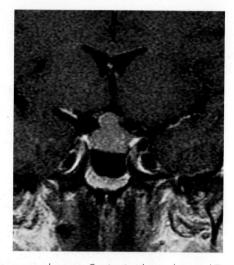

Fig. 2.13 Pituitary macroadenoma. Contrast enhanced coronal TI scan. A uniformly enhancing tumour is arising from the pituitary fossa and abutting the optic chasm.

Cerebral infarction (Figs 2.14–2.16)

The appearances are identical whether due to thrombosis or embolus. The main indication for CT is to exclude haemorrhage prior to anti-coagulant therapy.

■ Normal scan: may be seen if scanning is within 24 h of onset of symptoms.

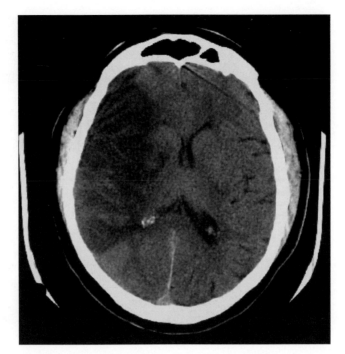

Fig. 2.14 Right middle cerebral artery infarction. Unenhanced CT.

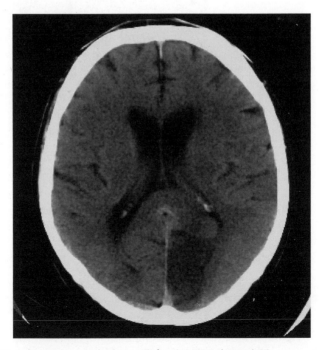

Fig. 2.15 Left posterior cerebral artery infarction. Unenhanced CT.

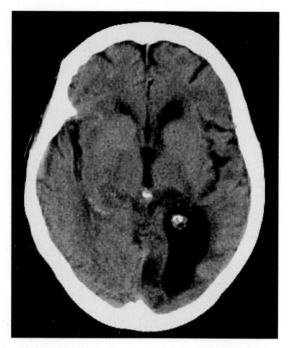

Fig. 2.16 Chronic infarct. Low density is seen in the left occipital lobe and there is enlargement of the adjacent lateral ventricle following an infarct at this site several years previously. Unenhanced CT.

- Acute infarct: ill-defined area of mildly reduced density in the region of a cerebral vessel. Often wedge-shaped. Little or no mass effect.
- Subacute infarct: over the next few weeks the area becomes more well defined and lower in density. Mass effect due to oedema is maximal at one week and thereafter decreases.
- Chronic infarct: very low density, with atrophy of the affected cortex and dilatation of the adjacent ventricle (Fig. 2.16).

  Further imaging:

- *As for TIAs* if there has been a full recovery and endarterectomy is contemplated.
- *Follow-up CT scans* may be indicated if condition deteriorates (e.g. due to extension of infarct or haemorrhage).
- *MRI* is more sensitive than CT in the first 24 h, due to its ability to detect oedema. However, it rarely proves clinically necessary.

Intracerebral haemorrhage (Fig. 2.17)

This most commonly occurs in hypertensive patients. It may also complicate arteriovenous malformations. Fresh haemorrhage is readily seen on an unenhanced CT.

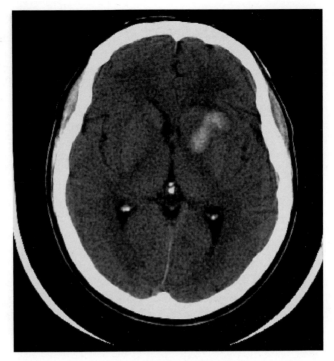

Fig. 2.17 Acute intracerebral haemorrhage. Unenhanced CT.

- Fresh blood: high-density (white) collection, usually in the basal ganglia, cerebellum or brainstem.
- Mass effect: dependent on the size of the haematoma and associated oedema.

Further imaging:

- *Cerebral angiography/MRA* if an underlying AVM is suspected.
- *Follow-up scans* as dictated by the condition of the patient.

EPILEPSY/FITTING

As with headache, most patients with epilepsy do not have a structural abnormality seen on CT scan. However, if there are any features to suggest this (e.g. residual signs after the fit) then scanning is appropriate. Additional features in the history will help determine which of the following possible underlying causes is most likely. Remember that a patient who is actively fitting will require sedating.

- Brain tumour: see p. 10.
- Encephalitis: see p. 7.
- Meningitis: see p. 7.
- Stroke: see p. 12.
- Trauma: see p. 19.

■ Arteriovenous malformation: this may not be visible on unenhanced CT unless there is calcification of the vessel wall(s). Contrast enhancement may reveal a serpiginous appearance. May also present with acute haemorrhage (see p. 16).

Further imaging:

■ Depends on the underlying cause.

MULTIPLE SCLEROSIS

The reader will be familiar with the various ways in which this condition can present. Although CT *may* show plaques of demyelination (low-density lesions with variable contrast enhancement) MRI is considerably more sensitive (Fig. 2.18) and is the investigation of choice. Plaques are seen as foci of high signal up to 3 cm in diameter (but usually ~ 1 cm), particularly around the lateral ventricles and in the spinal cord. However, these high signal foci are nonspecific and are often due to ischaemia. Furthermore, they are a frequent incidental finding in patients without any suggestion of demyelination, and are sometimes termed UBOs (unidentified bright objects). Their presence on an MRI must be closely correlated with the clinical situation before a label of MS is given.

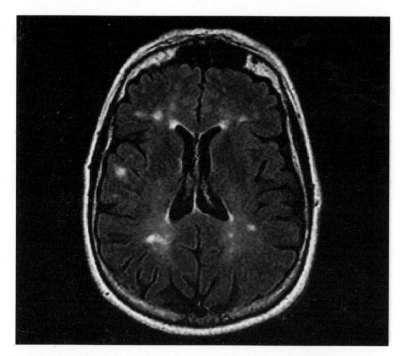

Fig. 2.18 Multiple sclerosis. Multiple high-signal foci due to plaques of demyelination. FLAIR sequence MRI.

COMA

The history will dictate the need for imaging. Where no history is available, metabolic causes of coma *must* be excluded or corrected before considering a CT; the last place for a uraemic patient with a high potassium to be is in a CT scanner. In the absence of trauma the commonest intracranial causes of coma are massive stroke and subarachnoid haemorrhage, the CT features of which are described above.

TRAUMA

Skull X-ray following trauma is probably *the* most overused radiological investigation. With the exception of confirming the presence of a depressed skull fracture, itself an indication to CT, it should not alter the management of a head-injured patient. This is because a normal skull X-ray *in no way* excludes serious intracranial injury; indeed most patients with subdural haematoma and many with extradural haematoma do *not* have a skull fracture; X-raying such patients does nothing except add expense and delay. (If you want to know what is inside a box you do not photograph the box!)

Correct clinical assessment is the key to selecting those patients who need a CT scan:

Absolute and relative indications for CT head scan following trauma

Absolute
- Decreased level of consciousness
- Focal neurological symptoms or signs
- Seizures
- Depressed fracture/penetrating injury

Relative
- Persisting or severe headache
- Vomiting
- Temporary loss of consciousness
- Amnesia

Notwithstanding the comments above look for the following on the skull X-rays:

- *Skull fracture* (Fig. 2.19): linear lucency in the skull vault. Absence of both branching and a sclerotic border help to distinguish from vessel markings, but can be very difficult.
- Depressed skull fracture (Fig. 2.20): overlapping bone edges cause dense opacity which does not immediately resemble a fracture. A tangential view shows it to best effect.

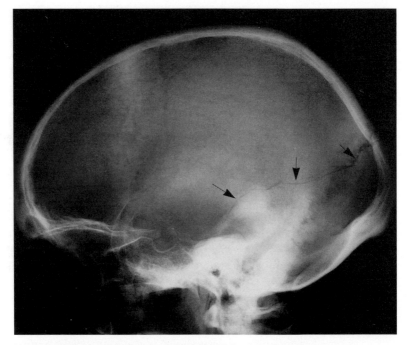

Fig. 2.19 Skull fracture (arrows). Lateral skull X-ray.

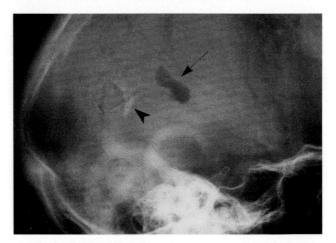

Fig. 2.20 Depressed skull fracture. Lateral skull X-ray. Note that the fracture is only visible as a dense line (arrowhead), due to the overlapping bone. Note also the presence of intracranial air (arrow).

■ Fluid level in sphenoid sinus: due to bleeding from a skull base fracture.

■ Cervical spine injury: but if this is suspected clinically then formal cervical spine views are mandatory.

On a CT scan the following should be looked for.

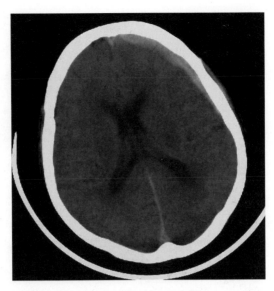

Fig. 2.21 Acute subdural haematoma. Unenhanced CT.

Acute subdural haematoma (Fig. 2.21)

This follows venous bleeding, often in the *absence* of skull fracture. They are invariably secondary to severe trauma and carry a poor prognosis.

■ Subdural collection: crescent-shaped high-density (i.e. white) collection between brain and inner skull vault.
■ Mass effect: proportional to the size of the collection.

Chronic subdural haematoma (Fig. 2.22)

The clinical situation is very different to acute subdural haematoma; these are usually seen in elderly patients and alcoholics with a history of recurrent falls, and their prognosis is much better. They are often bilateral. They too are seen as a crescentic-shaped collection extending along the cerebral surface, but they are intermediate or low in density depending on their age (>14 days are usually low density). When intermediate, their density may be exactly the same as brain, which makes them much less obvious. This is especially so when bilateral; look for medial displacement of both lateral ventricles. Acute bleeding within a chronic haematoma causes gravitational layering of different density collections (fresh, high-density blood below the low-density collection).

Extradural haematoma (Fig. 2.23)

This is usually due to meningeal artery bleeding following more significant trauma, often but not always associated with skull fracture.

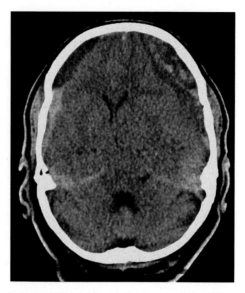

Fig. 2.22 Bilateral chronic subdural haematomas complicated by recurrent acute haemorrhage. Note the layering of fresh blood (white) below the low-density chronic (dark grey) haematoma. Note also the mass effect causing compression and displacement of the ventricles.

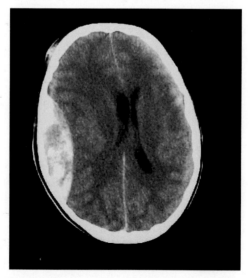

Fig. 2.23 Acute extradural haematoma, unenhanced CT. Note the biconvex shape and the significant mass effect.

- Extradural collection: biconvex high-density collection between the brain and skull vault.
- Mass effect: more significant than subdural bleeds, since high pressure, arterial bleeding.
- Cerebral contusions: frequently associated.

Cerebral contusion (Fig. 2.24)

This may be seen in isolation or in association with other intracranial injuries.

■ Contusion: fresh blood within the cerebral cortex extending to

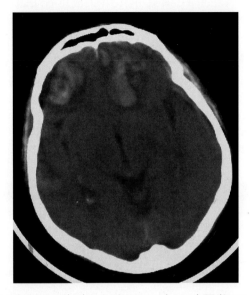

Fig. 2.24 Traumatic intracerebral contusions, unenhanced CT. (Same patient as Fig. 2.22.)

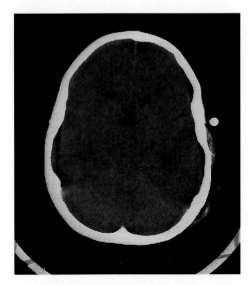

Fig. 2.25 Diffuse cerebral oedema, unenhanced CT. Severe trauma (RTA). The third ventricle and CSF space around the brainstem are completely effaced. (Compare with normal CT – Fig. 2.1.) The patient died the following day.

the inner skull vault. May correspond to the site of trauma or be on the contralateral side ('contra-coux').

Intracerebral haematoma

This is a localized collection of high-density blood within the cerebral or cerebellar cortex, more well defined than contusions, and does not extend to the skull vault. Mass effect is related to size.

Cerebral oedema (Fig. 2.25)

This occurs in relation to the above injuries or diffusely without associated focal haematoma. Diffuse cerebral oedema is indicated by effacement of the cerebral sulci and CSF-containing cisterns around the brainstem. This usually indicates diffuse axonal injury and a very poor prognosis.

Key points

- Skull X-rays are usually unhelpful in trauma, and may be falsely reassuring. They are very rarely indicated otherwise.
- Comatose patients should have metabolic derangement excluded before requesting CT scan.
- Acute infarction may not be evident on an initial CT scan.
- CT remains the investigation of choice following trauma or for suspected intracranial haemorrhage.
- MRI is very sensitive at detecting demyelination and encephalitis which are frequently associated with normal CT, but the MRI appearances of demyelination are nonspecific and often seen in normal patients.

The spine

3

IMAGING TECHNIQUES

Plain X-rays (Fig. 3.1)

AP and lateral views are obtained. Lateral views of the thoracic and lumbar spine are usually performed with the patient lying on their side. However, following trauma the patient is left supine to avoid causing spinal cord injury; the film is obtained using a 'horizontal beam', which is written on the film. This lateral view is invariably of poorer quality, but should allow vertebral body alignment and height to be assessed. Oblique views are occasionally helpful; in the cervical

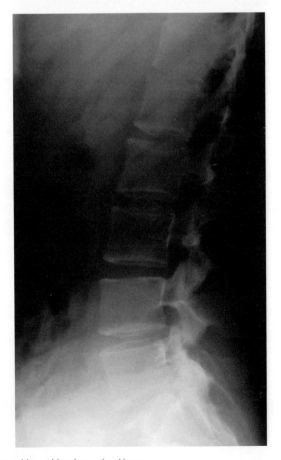

Fig. 3.1 Normal lateral lumbar spine X-ray.

spine they allow the exit foraminae to be assessed. In the lumbar spine they demonstrate spondylolysis defects of the laminae. X-ray of the lumbar spine carries a high radiation dose; equivalent to 120 CXRs.

Myelography

Water-soluble contrast is injected under fluoroscopic control into the thecal sac via a lumbar puncture. Spinal cord and nerve root compression can then be assessed. By tilting the patient the injected contrast can be run upwards to demonstrate the thoracic and cervical cord. An unpleasant procedure which has been rendered almost obsolete by CT and MRI.

CT (Fig. 3.2)

Thin slices (1–4 mm) are taken through the level of interest. Bony abnormalities are particularly well seen, e.g. fractures, spondylolysis, central canal stenosis. Disc herniation can usually be demonstrated, but the spinal cord is not well visualized.

MRI (Fig. 3.3)

The entire spine can be imaged in sagittal section, supplemented by axial slices through areas of interest. This is the investigation of choice for assessing spinal cord pathology, nerve root compression and intevertebral disc herniation. Recurrent symptoms following spinal surgery are also best assessed by MRI, which can distinguish

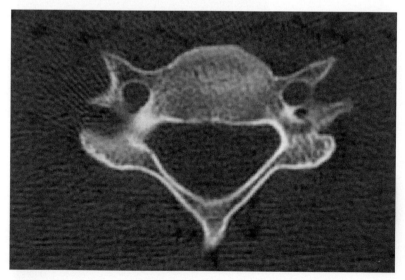

Fig. 3.2 Normal CT through an upper cervical vertebra. Note the beautiful bone detail.

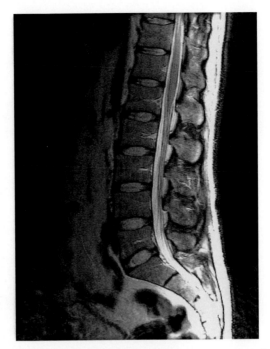

Fig. 3.3 Normal lumbar spine, MRI. Sagittal T2 sequence. Note the spinal cord and nerve roots (grey) surrounded by CSF (white).

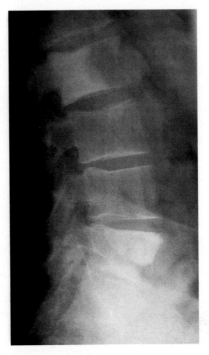

Fig. 3.4 Spinal metastases from prostate carcinoma, X-ray. Well-defined sclerotic deposits in the L1 and L4 vertebral bodies.

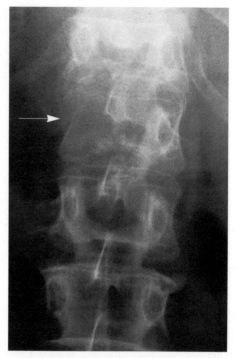

Fig. 3.5 Metastasis from breast carcinoma. The right pedicle of L2 is destroyed by a lytic metastasis (arrow).

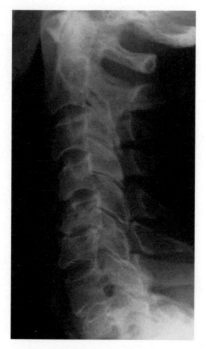

Fig. 3.6 Cervical spondylosis. Lateral X-ray showing disc space narrowing and osteophyte formation.

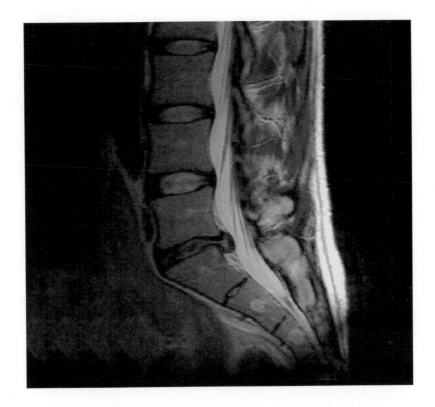

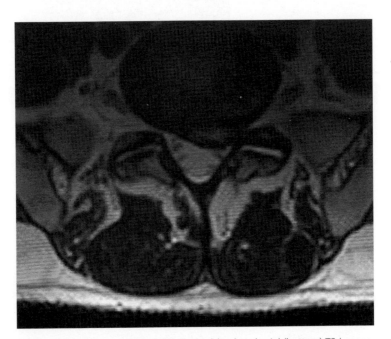

Fig. 3.7 Lumbar disc protrusion, MRI. Sagittal (top) and axial (bottom) T2 images showing a focal protrusion of the L5/S1 disc.

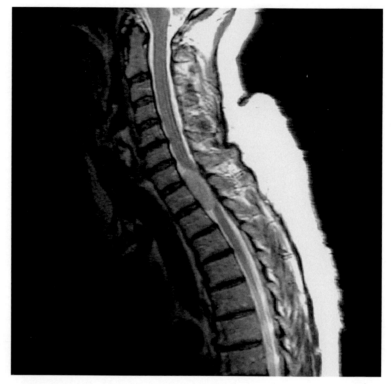

Fig. 3.8 Spinal cord compression on MRI (sagittal T2). The spinal cord is compressed by an intradural meningioma at the level of the T1 vertebral body.

between post-operative fibrosis and recurrent disc herniation. Bone detail is inferior to CT.

BACK PAIN

Acute back pain in the absence of neurological deficit is not an indication for X-ray except in the elderly, to exclude osteoporotic vertebral body collapse. Intervertebral disc herniation is not excluded by a normal X-ray. If symptoms persist for several weeks, or in the presence of neurological involvement (e.g. sensorimotor symptoms or sphincter disturbance) then CT or MRI is indicated.

Similarly, *chronic back pain* is not an indication for X-ray unless there is clinical concern about malignancy or infection (e.g. severe pain unrelieved by rest, weight loss, known primary neoplasm, systemic symptoms) (Figs 3.4, 3.5). In this group it is important to note that a normal X-ray does not exclude skeletal metastases, so isotope bone scan or MRI should then be performed. The same may be true of low-grade chronic infection, classically TB, where a high index of suspicion should be maintained in the presence of normal X-rays. Early follow-up films or MRI should be considered here.

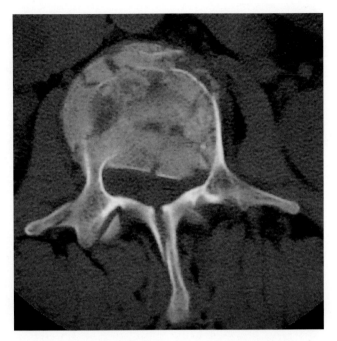

Fig. 3.9 CT scan showing a burst fracture of a lumbar vertebra. Fracture fragments have been displaced posteriorly to encroach on the spinal canal. Note that there are also fractures involving the right transverse and spinous processes.

NEUROLOGICAL SPINAL DISORDERS (SCIATICA, CERVICAL SPONDYLOSIS, SPINAL CORD COMPRESSION)

Since lumbar disc herniation may be present despite normal plain X-rays, it follows that when this diagnosis is suspected due to signs of nerve root entrapment, MRI is the investigation of choice. It enables visualization of the herniated disc itself and its effect on the adjacent nerve roots (Fig. 3.7).

Cervical spondylosis (Fig. 3.6) is also more reliably assessed by MRI than CT, although even MRI can be difficult because of artefacts caused by swallowing and arterial pulsations. Some centres continue to practice cervical myelography for this reason.

Acute spinal cord compression is one of the few indications for urgent MRI, which will usually identify the level and the cause (Fig. 3.8).

TRAUMA

Plain radiographs are indicated in the initial assessment. Depending on the severity of injury these may be technically difficult, and inferior in quality (see notes above regarding 'horizontal beam' radiographs).

CT is indicated if there is concern about a particular level following plain radiographs, or to visualize the full extent of a fracture which has been demonstrated (Fig. 3.9). It can help to assess stability or otherwise of a given fracture, but not invariably so since ligamentous disruption is not demonstrated.

MRI does not demonstrate fractures with the same detail as CT, but has the advantage of showing associated ligamentous, soft tissue and spinal cord injuries.

Key points

- Spinal metastases and infection are not visible on X-rays until there is significant bone destruction. Isotope bone scan or MRI are considerably more sensitive.
- Disc protrusions are not excluded by a normal X-ray. MRI is required.
- Acute nontraumatic back pain is not an indication for X-ray unless there is suspicion of spontaneous vertebral body collapse or malignancy.
- Back pain without neurological symptoms is not an indication for MRI.

The chest

4

IMAGING TECHNIQUES

Chest X-ray

In a well patient this is performed *erect PA* (Fig. 4.1); the patient stands with the film cassette in contact with the anterior chest wall and exposure is made at peak inspiration. Thus the X-ray beam passes from *p*osterior to *a*nterior. Radiation dose is minimal; equivalent to 3 days natural background radiation.

In patients unable to stand the film has to be performed *AP sitting* (Fig. 4.2), with the cassette in contact with the posterior chest wall. This has a number of effects on the appearance of the X-ray, which should not be misinterpreted as being due to abnormality. The heart may appear enlarged beyond the normal cardiothoracic ratio (CTR – the ratio of heart size to chest diameter) of 0.5. Similarly the hila appear larger and the mediastinum appears wider. The lungs may not be well visualized, especially if the patient is unable to take a full

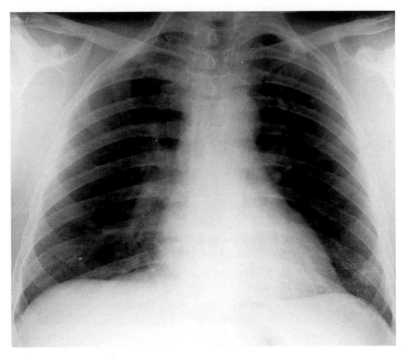

Fig. 4.1 Normal PA CXR.

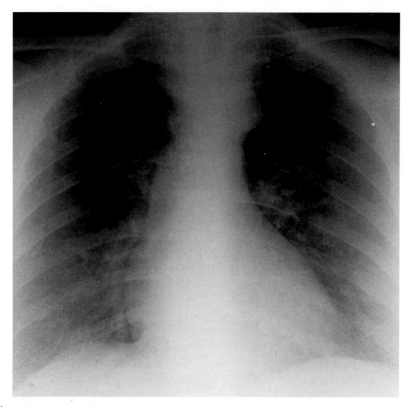

Fig. 4.2 Normal AP CXR. Note the apparent cardiac enlargement and position of scapulae over the chest.

breath in. When these effects are significant a PA film should always be performed once the patient's condition allows.

A *lateral CXR* (Fig. 4.3) is performed routinely with the PA film in some departments, whilst in others it is performed to further evaluate or localize an abnormality seen on the frontal view. It also helps clarify lobar consolidation and collapse.

Occasionally a chest X-ray is performed *AP supine* (e.g. ITU). Apart from the aforementioned effects, note that the diaphragm will be elevated. Also the appearance of disease is altered; pleural effusion fluid will pool posteriorly, causing hazy opacification of the whole lung (Fig. 4.4); the signs of pneumoperitoneum and pneumothorax become subtle, or may be absent. *Lateral decubitus films* may then be helpful; these are taken with the patient lying on his/her left side and can demonstrate very small volumes of free air (<5 ml).

Patients unable to attend the X-ray department may be imaged on the ward using a *portable X-ray machine.* Try to avoid requesting this on anything but the sickest patients; the films obtained are never as good as from a departmental machine and they are an inefficient use of radiographer time.

Note that a poor inspiration will cause haziness at the bases due to

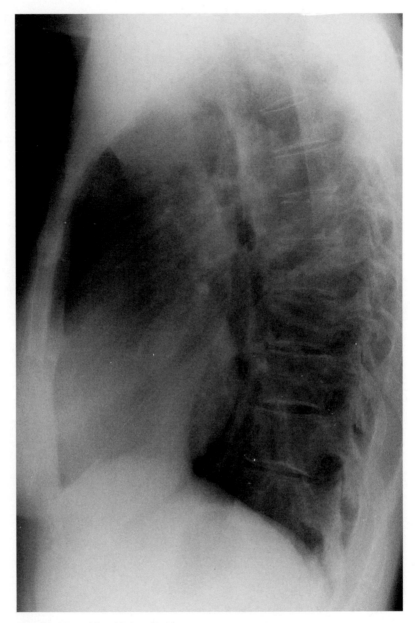

Fig. 4.3 Normal lateral chest X-ray.

atelectasis as well as apparent cardiac enlargement and mediastinal widening (Fig. 4.5); this should not be mistaken for disease. On a well-inspired film the anterior ends of the first six ribs should be seen overlying the lungs. Other potential pitfalls are breast implants, which can mimic lower zone abnormality (Fig. 4.6) and the chest deformity pes excavatum, which mimics R middle lobe consolidation (Fig. 4.7).

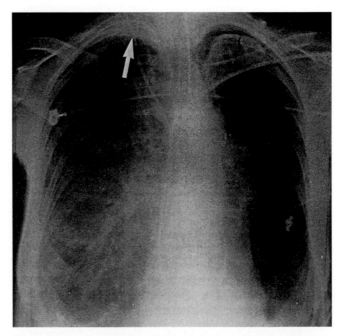

Fig. 4.4 Pleural effusion in the supine patient. In this supine patient a right-sided effusion produces a veil-like opacity in the lower chest through which preserved lung vessels can be seen. In addition the diaphragm is ill-defined, the costophrenic angle blunted and there is a typical apical cap (arrow). (Courtesy of Grainger & Alison, *Diagnostic Radiology* 3rd edit., Churchill Livingstone.)

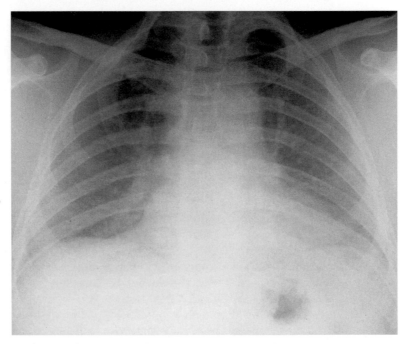

Fig. 4.5 Effect of a poor inspiration on CXR appearance. Same patient as Fig. 4.1, taken 5 min before.

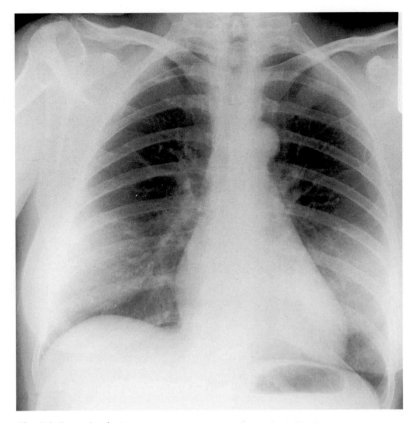

Fig. 4.6 Breast implants.

Analysing a chest X-ray

Try to develop a checklist which you work through every time you view a CXR. It does not matter what sequence you use; what matters is that you remember to use it every time. The main reason abnormalities are missed is failure to use such a routine.

■ *Heart*: size, contour, position within the chest.
■ *Lungs*: focal abnormalities are usually obvious. Compare one lung with the other; are they equal volume and equal density? Are the pulmonary vessels symmetrical?
■ *Mediastinum*: is it displaced to one side? Is there a mass within it ?
■ *Review areas*: these are where radiologists earn their money; the areas where abnormalities are missed if not specifically looked for. Look *under the diaphragm* for evidence of free intraperitoneal air, *behind the heart* where lung masses frequently hide (Fig. 4.8). Look at the *hila*: are they normal size? If enlarged is it due to lymph node or pulmonary artery enlargement? (It is not always possible to tell.) Look at the *apices* for pancoast tumours and at the *bones* for rib and spine lesions. In a female always check the *breasts* for evidence of mastectomy.

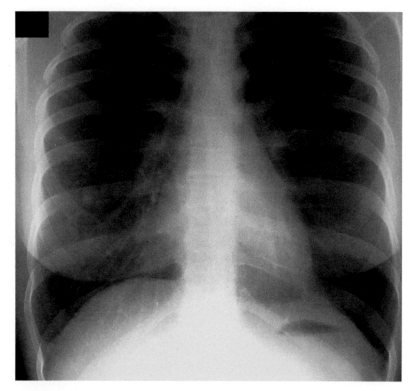

Fig. 4.7 Pes excavatum. This chest deformity causes poor definition of the right heart border, thus mimicking right middle lobe consolidation. The configuration of the ribs (horizontal posterior aspects, sloping anterior aspects) is a clue. If in doubt examine the patient!

CT of thorax (Fig. 4.9)

The patient lies supine or prone in the scanner. The thorax is scanned in slices of varying thickness, depending on the suspected pathology. Newer machines ('spiral CT') can scan the whole chest in one breath-hold. Radiation dose is significant; 4 years background radiation (i.e. 400 CXRs).

The lungs, mediastinum and thoracic skeleton are well visualized by altering the window settings. Parenchymal abnormalities not visible on a plain CXR can be seen. Central neoplasms and lymphadenopathy are also well demonstrated. Intravenous contrast allows visualization of vascular abnormalities such as aortic dissection and pulmonary embolism, and helps to differentiate hilar and mediastinal masses from blood vessels. *HRCT* (high-resolution CT) involves thin slices (usually 1 mm thickness at 1 cm intervals) and demonstrates the lung parenchyma in exquisite detail.

Ultrasound

The ultrasound probe is applied directly to the chest wall; no radiation.

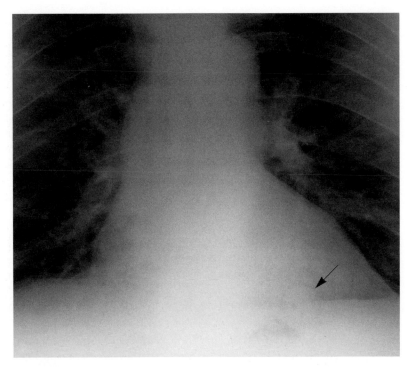

Fig. 4.8 A small lung opacity projected through the heart shadow is easily missed (arrow). In this case it was due to a lung metastasis.

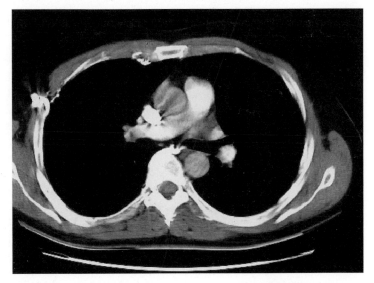

Fig. 4.9 Normal contrast-enhanced CT of thorax, at level of right main pulmonary artery.

Echocardiography demonstrates the heart in considerable detail; ventricular function and valvular disease are well visualized.

Pleural and pericardial effusions are well visualized; ultrasound can distinguish between loculated and free pleural fluid. Chest wall abnormalities are also well seen. Consolidated or collapsed lung is seen, but aerated lung and mediastinum are not visualized.

Radionuclide studies

A ventilation-perfusion (VQ) scan is performed for suspected pulmonary embolism. In the ventilation phase the patient breathes radiolabelled gas, and in the perfusion phase an IV injection of radio-labelled microspheres is administered. The patient is then scanned on a gamma camera. Radiation dose is equivalent to 7 months background radiation (60 CXRs).

Cardiac isotope studies allow demonstration of myocardial ischaemia (thallium- and technetium-labelled pyrophosphate scans) and ventricular function (labelled RBC scan). The radiation dose for a thallium myocardium scan dose is equivalent to 9 years background radiation (900 CXRs).

MRI of thorax

This is of limited use in pulmonary disease, since the long scan times mean it is susceptible to significant artefacts from cardiac motion and respiration. Cardiac MRI can demonstrate valvular and ischaemic heart disease, cardiac masses and congenital defects, and its use in these areas is likely to increase.

Angiography

Pulmonary angiography is indicated for suspected pulmonary embolism (PE) following an indeterminate VQ scan, although many departments now perform contrast-enhanced spiral CT instead. A 5–7f catheter is inserted into the femoral vein under local anaesthesia and passed up the IVC, through the R heart chambers and into the pulmonary artery. Images are obtained whilst contrast is rapidly injected into the pulmonary arteries. The main complication is cardiac arrhythmia as the catheter passes through the heart. Pulmonary oedema may also be provoked. However, the risks are often overstated; the overall mortality is still less than 1 in 1000.

Coronary angiography is indicated for the investigation of ischaemic heart disease. A catheter is inserted via the femoral or brachial artery under local anaesthetic, and passed retrogradely to the aortic root and into the L ventricle. Contrast injection into the L ventricle allows assessment of LV function and demonstrates mitral and aortic valve disease. Selective injections into the R and L coronary arteries allows demonstration of stenoses and occlusions. The main complications are cardiac arrhythmia, coronary artery dissection or occlusion and CVA due to embolization. Overall mortality is less than 1 in 1000. Coronary artery angioplasty involves balloon dilatation of stenoses performed via a femoral approach under local anaesthesia. This avoids or defers the need for CABG, and may also be performed on CABG stenoses. Cardiac arrhythmias are more common than during simple diagnostic angiography. The risk of coronary artery dissection and occlusion is also significantly higher, so the patient is usually consented for emergency CABG should the need arise. Mortality rates depend very much on case complexity, but are usually between 1 and 2%. Aortography is performed using the same technique and is indicated for the demonstration of traumatic aortic rupture and (depending on local policy) aortic dissection.

BREATHLESSNESS

The chest X-ray should be the first radiological investigation performed in the assessment of the breathless patient. The following conditions should be looked for.

Cardiac failure (Figs 4.10, 4.11)

Chest X-ray features, in order of increasing severity:

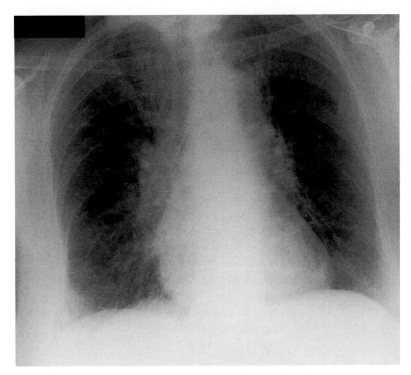

Fig. 4.10 Acute cardiac failure following myocardial infarction. The heart is not enlarged, but there is perihilar venous distension and there are septal lines in the lower zones. The patient had an acute myocardial infarction.

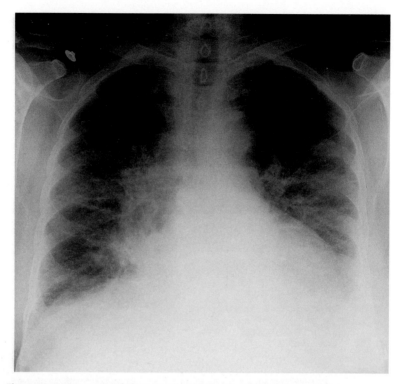

Fig. 4.11 Severe cardiac failure. Cardiomegaly, pleural effusions, perihilar venous distension and interstitial lines.

- Cardiomegaly: such that the cardiothoracic on a PA film exceeds the normal 0.5. In mild cases this may be the only CXR abnormality.
- Distension of upper lobe veins: their diameter equals or exceeds that of the lower lobe vessels. This indicates pulmonary venous hypertension.
- Kerley B lines: horizontal lines at the periphery of the bases due to interstitial oedema.
- Pleural effusions: usually bilateral, but may be asymmetrical or unilateral if the patient has been lying on one side, or if there is pre-existing lung disease (e.g. COPD).
- Alveolar oedema: seen as 'air space shadowing' which is identical in appearance to infective consolidation, but differs in distribution; classically a bilateral perihilar distribution is seen ('bat's wing') but in severe cases it may be throughout the lungs, mimicking diffuse pneumonia.

Further imaging:

- *Repeat CXRs* to follow disease progression/response to therapy.
- *Echocardiography* to assess ventricular function and valvular disease.

■ *Cardiac isotope studies* depending on local policy.
■ *Coronary angiography* if a candidate for CABG.

Chest infection

Immunocompetent patients (Figs 4.12–4.14)

In the early stages the chest X-ray may be normal. Thereafter infective consolidation is seen as:

■ Air space shadowing: localized distribution, lobar or segmental. 'Air bronchograms' represent air-filled bronchi surrounded by fluid-filled alveoli.
■ Pleural effusion: may be associated. Invariably unilateral.
■ Hilar lymphadenopathy: especially viral pneumonia and primary TB.
■ Cavity formation: particularly with TB, staphylococcal, aspergillosis and klebsiella infections.

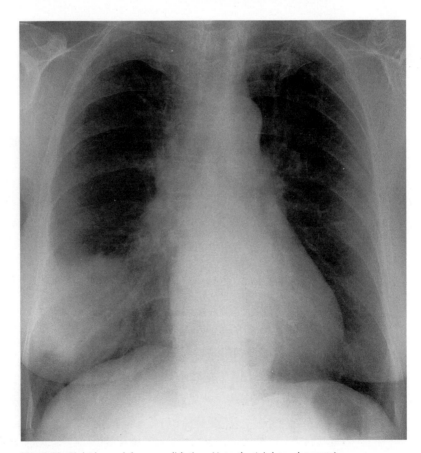

Fig. 4.12 Right lower lobe consolidation. Note the 'air bronchogram'.

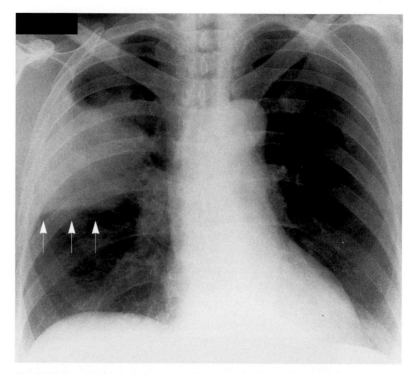

Fig. 4.13 Dense right upper lobe consolidation. Note how the opacification abuts the horizontal fissure inferiorly (arrows).

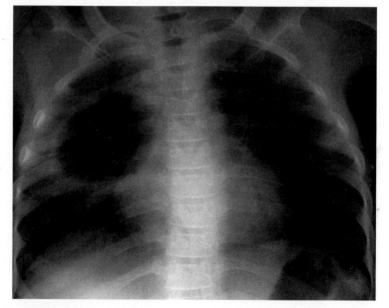

Fig. 4.14 Cavitating pneumonia. A large cavity is seen in the right upper lobe in a child with tuberculosis.

Further imaging:

- *Repeat CXRs* to follow disease progression. Resolution of CXR signs is slow in the elderly, so allow 1 week per decade of life before performing a repeat film. Other imaging is not required unless there is evidence of an underlying cause, e.g. carcinoma bronchus.
- *CT thorax* if the diagnosis is uncertain or a proximal bronchial tumour is suspected.

Immunocompromised patients

This is most commonly due to haematological malignancy and associated chemotherapy, immunosuppressive treatment used in transplant patients and AIDS. Immunosuppression alters the host response to conventional infections and makes the patient susceptible to 'atypical infections' by organisms which do not usually cause disease. These include *Pneumocystis carinii* (PCP) (Fig. 4.15), *Mycobacterium tuberculosis, Candida albicans, Herpes* and *Cytomegaloviruses.*

The threshold for requesting a CXR in immunosuppressed patients should therefore be lowered. However, it is important to recognize that such infections may be associated with almost any CXR appearance, including normal. Mixed infections are also common,

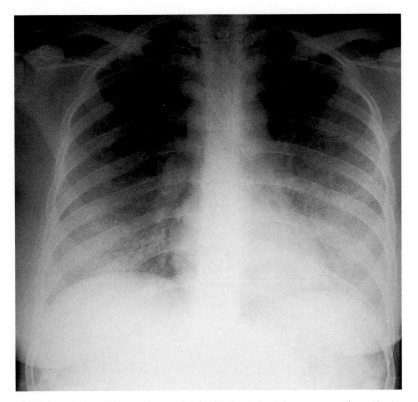

Fig. 4.15 PCP in AIDS. Hazy interstitial shadowing in both lower zones. The patient died shortly afterwards.

and the presence of noninfective pathology such as localised primary disease (e.g. in lymphoma and leukaemia) or Kaposi's sarcoma (in AIDS). It is therefore quite impossible to offer a microbiological diagnosis on the basis of the CXR appearances. In a patient known to be immunosuppressed, clinical suspicion of infection should, regardless of the CXR appearance, prompt vigorous attempts to isolate the organism by means such as bronchoscopic biopsy. The main value of the CXR is to follow the progress of the disease.

It also follows that if a patient with a clinical chest infection has widespread severe changes on the CXR, an underlying immunosuppressive condition should be considered.

Pulmonary embolism

In the absence of pre-existing lung disease the CXR is usually normal, but look for:

- Localized oligaemia: seen as increased lucency in the affected area.
- Increased pulmonary artery diameter: due to intraluminal thrombus.
- Localized consolidation: in subacute cases. Varied appearance but wedge-shaped peripheral consolidation is very suggestive of underlying infarction.

Further imaging:

- *Ventilation-perfusion (V/Q) scan.* If normal this excludes PE with >95% sensitivity. If there are two or more unmatched perfusion defects, this confirms PE with 90–95% sensitivity. Other appearances are less specific; an 'indeterminate' scan is associated with a 30–40% probability of PE, and should lead to further investigation. Note that patients with COPD frequently have indeterminate scans.
- *Pulmonary angiogram.* Current 'gold standard'. Emboli are seen as filling defects within the opacified pulmonary arteries (Fig. 4.16).
- *CT thorax.* As an alternative to pulmonary angiography. Spiral CT scanner required. Intravenous contrast enhanced slices through the pulmonary arteries may demonstrate the filling defect(s) (Fig. 4.17). Will also demonstrate other pathologies.
- *Lower-limb doppler ultrasound/venography.* If pulmonary angiography is contraindicated. If normal then the patient is unlikely to be at risk of further PE (but pelvic vein thrombus cannot be excluded).

Asthma

CXR appearances:

- Hyperinflated lungs: The posterior aspect of the 11th ribs is visible above the diaphragm, which is flattened.

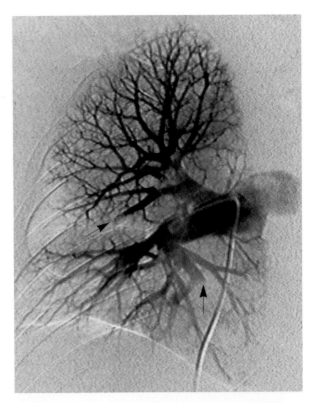

Fig. 4.16 Pulmonary embolism on pulmonary angiography. A catheter is positioned in the right pulmonary artery. Note the abrupt occlusion of some of the arteries by thrombus (arrows) with no contrast enhancement of the vessel distally.

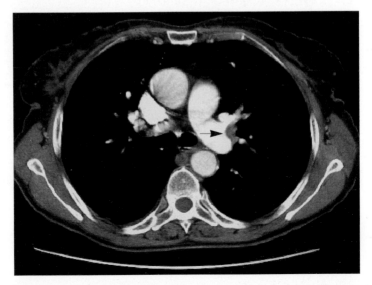

Fig. 4.17 Pulmonary embolus, left pulmonary artery (arrow). Contrast-enhanced spiral CT.

■ Infective consolidation: may have provoked an acute attack.
■ Lobar collapse: due to mucus plugging. See pp 53–56 for the different appearances.
■ Pneumothorax: unusual, but should always be carefully looked for.

Further imaging:

■ In the absence of the latter two complications this is not indicated.

Pneumothorax (Fig. 4.18)

CXR appearances:

■ Lung does not extend to the periphery of the chest: look carefully for lung edge, especially at the apices (easy to miss if the lungs are otherwise normal).
■ Air in pleural space: absent lung markings.
■ Mediastinal shift: towards the opposite side. This indicates a tension pneumothorax, a medical emergency requiring

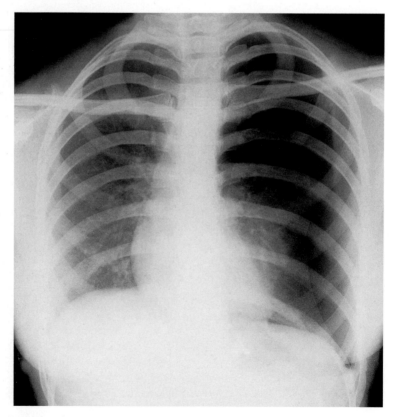

Fig. 4.18 Left pneumothorax. Note the shift of the heart and the mediastinum to the right.

immediate drainage. (NB: if this is suspected on clinical examination *do not delay treatment* to obtain a CXR.)

Further imaging:

■ *CXR in expiration or in lateral decubitus position* (with suspected side uppermost) will show a small pneumothorax not visible on the standard view, but is only occasionally warranted.
■ *Follow-up CXRs* after the insertion of a chest drain to check for drain position and lung re-expansion (but daily films rarely justified).

Chronic airways disease (Figs 4.19, 4.20)

Most patients have a combination of chronic bronchitis and emphysema. The CXR features will thus be a combination of the two:

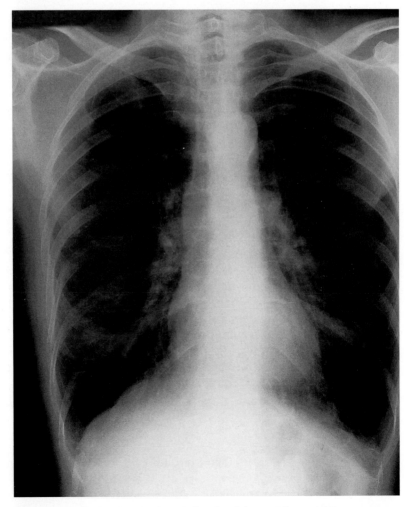

Fig. 4.19 COAD: the lungs are hyperinflated and there are increased bronchovascular markings.

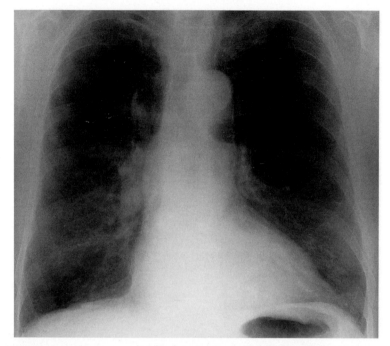

Fig. 4.20 COAD. The lungs are hyperinflated causing flattening of the diaphragm. The left upper zone is hyperlucent due to emphysematous disease.

- Hyperexpanded lungs: flattened hemidiaphragms; the posterior part of the 11th ribs is visible above the diaphragm.
- Bullae: rounded, thin-walled areas of reduced markings. They can simulate a pneumothorax, especially if apical.
- Bronchial wall thickening: linear shadows.
- Scarring and fibrosis: dense linear shadows.
- Super-added consolidation: accounting for acute deterioration. Difficult to diagnose without comparison with previous films.
- Cor pulmonale: the R ventricle and main pulmonary arteries increase in size due to the pulmonary arterial hypertension which occurs with chronic lung disease. The L heart border is prominent and the cardiac apex is elevated. Best assessed by comparison with previous films. Note that cardiac failure in this situation may occur without cardiomegaly.

NB: CXR may be *normal* even in the presence of clinically significant disease.

Further imaging:

- *Repeat CXRs* to follow resolution of superadded infection. At greater intervals to assess disease progression; look especially for evidence of developing cor pulmonale.
- *HRCT of thorax* demonstrates fibrosis much more sensitively. Complicating bronchial carcinoma more clearly demonstrated.

Will also differentiate bullae from pneumothorax when the CXR is equivocal.

Industrial lung disease (pneumoconiosis)

Although industrial exposure to inorganic dusts causes CXR abnormality, this does not necessarily account for breathlessness, or indeed any symptoms. However, coexistent chronic airways disease due to cigarette smoking is frequent, and will account for symptoms. The commonest appearance of simple coal workers' pneumoconiosis is of multiple small opacities throughout the lungs which may calcify; an appearance not unlike miliary TB. 'Complicated' pneumoconiosis is due to secondary fibrosis, and *is* responsible for breathlessness. Progressive massive fibrosis (PMF) occurs in <20% of coal miners, and causes marked fibrosis usually in both upper lobes (Fig. 4.22). The CXR shows dense upper zone masses, scarring and volume loss seen as elevation of the hila.

Further imaging:

■ *Repeat CXRs* will show progression of secondary fibrosis.
■ *HRCT of thorax* demonstrates fibrosis more sensitively. Asbestos-related pleural plaques and mesothelioma well seen, as is complicating bronchial carcinoma.

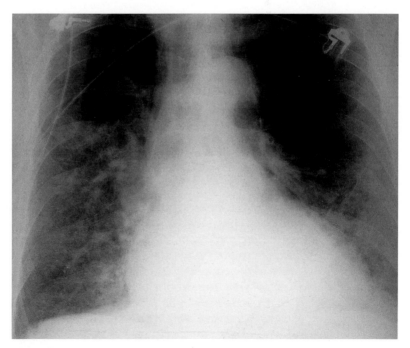

Fig. 4.21 COAD complicated by an infective exacerbation. Same patient as Fig. 4.20, showing super-added consolidation at both bases. Note the poor visualization of the left hemidiaphragm compared with Fig. 4.20.

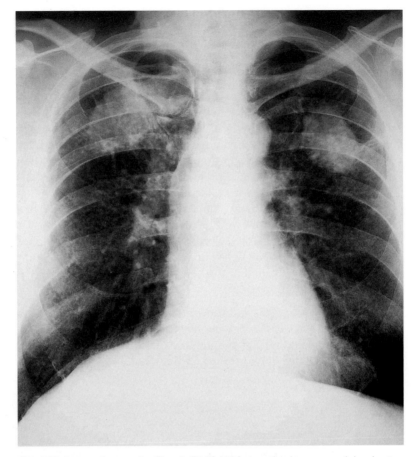

Fig. 4.22 Progressive massive fibrosis (PMF). Widespread pulmonary nodules due to pneumoconiosis complicated by bilateral apical fibrosis.

Pleural effusion (Fig. 4.23)

At least 175 ml of pleural fluid are needed to be seen on a PA film. A lateral decubitus film, with the suspected side down, is more sensitive; 75 ml will be visible.

■ Effusion fluid: seen as a dense collection in the costophrenic angle(s). The superior border usually curves up the side of the chest (the 'meniscus sign'). The chest X-ray appearance is altered by patient position; in the supine position fluid pools to cause haziness of the entire hemithorax (Fig. 4.4).

■ Mediastinal shift: towards the opposite side. If there is no shift despite the presence of a large effusion then associated lung collapse is usual, and is often due to underlying malignancy.

■ Underlying cause: not usually evident, but look for signs of cardiac failure, infection or malignancy. If there is a history of asbestos exposure, suspect an underlying mesothelioma, which is seen as an irregular pleural-based mass often encasing the entire lung.

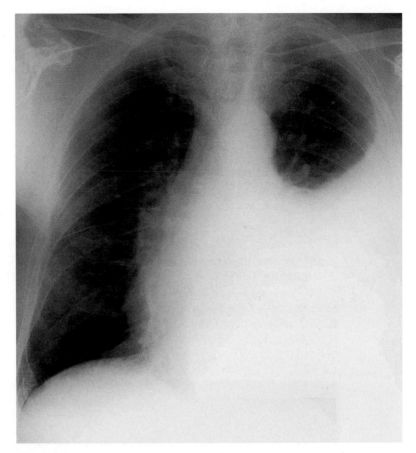

Fig. 4.23 Large pleural effusion.

Further imaging:

- *Repeat CXRs* to follow progression or response to treatment. After drainage procedures look to see if an underlying lesion is now visible and check for pneumothorax.
- *Ultrasound of thorax* will demonstrate very small effusions, and the presence of septations or loculations within them. Ultrasound guidance allows accurate drainage of fluid for diagnostic or therapeutic purposes.

Other imaging will depend on underlying cause.

Lobar collapse

If the remainder of the lungs is normal this may not result in significant breathlessness. However, in the presence of underlying lung disease collapse of a single lobe may cause severe clinical deterioration. The CXR appearances depend on the lobe affected, but common to all are:

■ Increased density: due to the collapsed lobe itself.
■ Volume loss: the amount depends on which lobe is affected. Causes variable 'rib crowding', mediastinal shift towards the affected side, elevation of hemidiaphragm, shift of hilum and interlobar fissures.
■ Compensatory hyperexpansion of other lobes: variable, depending on their normality; may completely fill the space created by the collapse. The CXR shows hyperlucency and spreading out of vascular markings.

Also look for evidence of an underlying lesion, especially bronchial carcinoma.

■ *RLL collapse* (Fig. 4.24): R basal density; depression of R hilum and horizontal fissure.
■ *RML collapse* (Fig. 4.25): the RML is small, so even complete collapse results in subtle signs. Poor definition of the R heart border may be the only sign on a PA film. The horizontal fissure may be depressed, but is often not visible. A lateral or lordotic view shows the increased density due to the collapsed lobe very clearly.
■ *RUL collapse* (Fig. 4.26): R upper zone density; elevation of R hilum and horizontal fissure.

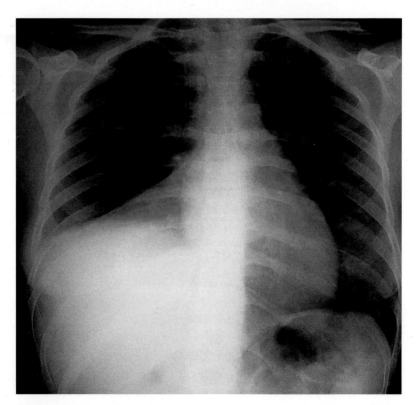

Fig. 4.24 Right lower lobe collapse.

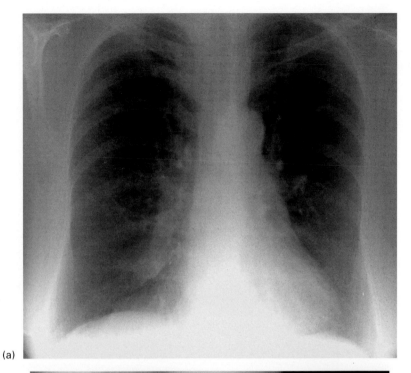

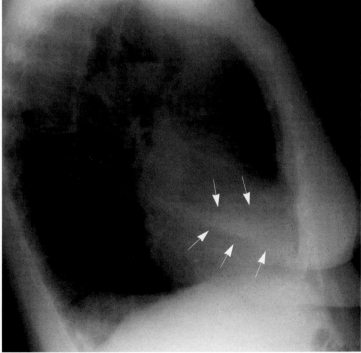

Fig. 4.25 Right middle lobe collapse. (a) PA CXR: the right heart border is poorly defined and there is depression of the right main bronchus. (b) The wedge-shaped density due to the collapsed lobe is easily seen on the lateral view (arrows).

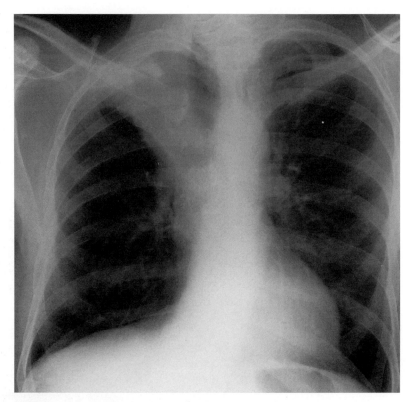

Fig. 4.26 Right upper lobe collapse.

- *LLL collapse* (Fig. 4.27): L lower zone density visible through the cardiac shadow. L hilum depressed.
- *LUL collapse* (Fig. 4.28): very different appearance to RUL collapse! The collapsed lobe is seen as a *hazy* density in the L upper zone; the appearance is easily confused with consolidation or pleural fluid/thickening. L hilar elevation is usually subtle or absent. A lateral view shows a density in the upper zone and anterior shift of the oblique fissure.

Further imaging:

- *Additional view CXRs* e.g. lateral or lordotic views for suspected RML collapse. Lateral view for suspected LUL collapse.
- *CT of thorax* to look for a central tumour as the underlying cause. Not necessary if bronchoscopy planned, but if a tumour is diagnosed may be indicated for staging.

Congenital heart disease

Severe congenital heart defects will usually be apparent clinically at or shortly after birth. They are beyond the scope of this text. Milder defects may not present until adult life.

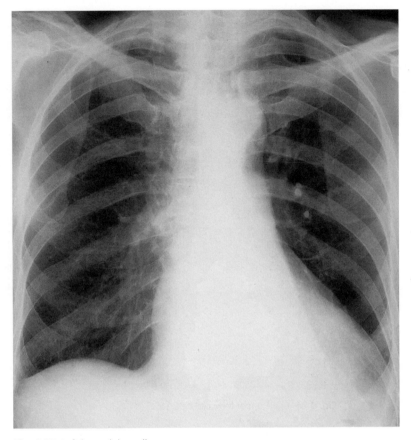

Fig. 4.27 Left lower lobe collapse.

- *Atrial septal defect (ASD)*: this is the commonest defect to present in adulthood. The CXR will only be abnormal when L to R flow through the defect is greater than twice aortic flow (i.e. pulmonary : systemic flow ratio >2 : 1). The heart enlarges due to R atrial and R ventricular enlargement; classically this causes a prominent R heart border and elevation of the cardiac apex. The main pulmonary arteries are also enlarged.
- *Ventricular septal defect (VSD)* (Fig. 4.29): large defects will present in the neonatal period. However small defects may not present until adult life. As with ASDs the CXR appearances will depend on the size of the defect, and degree of shunting through it. Cardiomegaly and pulmonary artery enlargement is again seen, such that differentiation between an ASD and a VSD is often not possible on plain film. However, L atrial enlargement does not occur in ASD, and therefore suggests a VSD.
- *Congenital aortic stenosis*: (Fig. 4.30): onset of symptoms is dependent on the severity of the stenosis. The CXR shows L ventricular enlargement, seen as prominence of the left heart

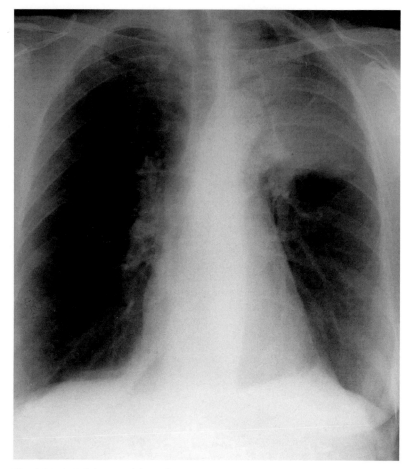

Fig. 4.28 CXR, left upper lobe collapse.

border with inferior displacement of the cardiac apex. Valvular calcification and post-stenotic dilatation of the ascending aorta may also be seen, and look for evidence of associated cardiac failure. Note that pulmonary vascularity is normal, since there is no shunt.

■ *Coarctation of the aorta*: narrowing of the aortic isthmus, the site of insertion of the fetal ductus arteriosus, just distal to the origin of the L subclavian artery. Usually presents in young adulthood with hypertension, but breathlessness occurs if there is secondary cardiac failure. The CXR shows L ventricular enlargement, aortic dilatation proximal and distal to the narrowing ('figure 3 aorta') and bilateral rib notching. Again pulmonary vascularity is normal.

Further imaging:

■ *Serial CXRs* to look for complications, particularly cardiac failure.
■ *Echocardiography*: septal defects are well seen, and differentiation

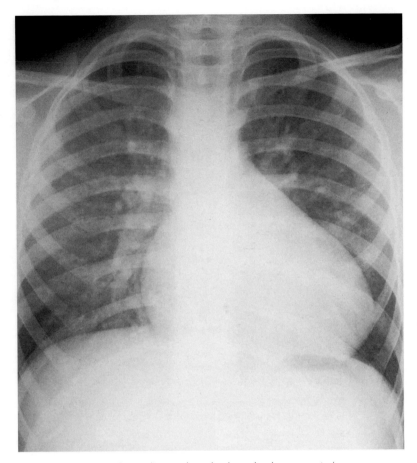

Fig. 4.29 VSD. Note the cardiomegaly and enlarged pulmonary arteries.

between different types (e.g. primum and secundum ASDs) is possible. Doppler allows measurement of pressure gradients across valvular stenoses, which helps in deciding whether surgery is indicated.

■ *Angiography* will demonstrate associated abnormalities, which are not uncommon, and allows assessment of the coronary arteries prior to surgery.

■ *MRI* may demonstrate complex defects very elegantly, and its use is likely to increase as new imaging sequences become available.

CHEST PAIN

The first imaging investigation should be a plain chest X-ray, PA erect if the patient's condition allows; otherwise an AP sitting film. Conditions to consider are as follows.

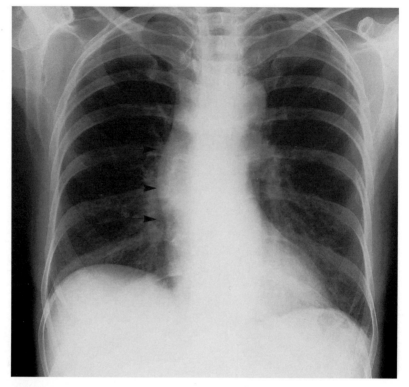

Fig. 4.30 Aortic stenosis. There is post-stenotic dilatation of the ascending aorta (arrows). The heart is normal in size.

Ischaemic heart disease

An acute angina attack or myocardial infarction is frequently associated with an entirely normal CXR. However, look for the following:

- Cardiac failure: see p. 41. But note that cardiac failure secondary to acute MI is often associated with a normal heart size (Fig. 4.10). Overwhelming cardiac failure implies massive infarction or (rarely) ruptured chorda tendinae or ventricular septum.
- Median sternotomy wires and CABG clips: as evidence of previous cardiac surgery.
- Ventricular aneurysm (Fig. 4.31): invariably L ventricle. Bulging of the cardiac apex, frequently shows curvilinear calcification.

Further imaging:

- *Echocardiography* will assess ventricular function (ejection fraction) and detect valve disease.
- *Coronary angiography* detects coronary artery stenoses and occlusions. Angioplasty dilatation of suitable stenoses prevents or delays the need for CABG.
- *Isotope scanning*: thallium scan detects areas of reversible ischaemia; *labelled RBC scan* to assess ventricular function; *Tc-*

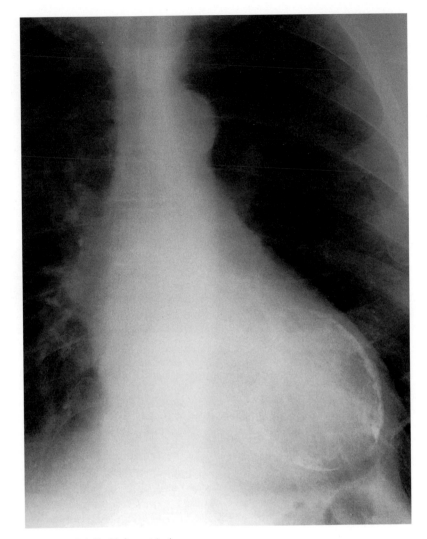

Fig. 4.31 Calcified left ventricular aneurysm.

pyrophosphate scan detects acute infarcts (but only after several hours).

Aortic dissection (Fig. 4.32)

CXR is nonspecific in 75% of cases, but look for:

- Mediastinal widening: often difficult to assess, especially on an AP film and without previous films for comparison.
- Pleural effusion: due to blood in pleural space.
- Localized dilatation of aortic knuckle.

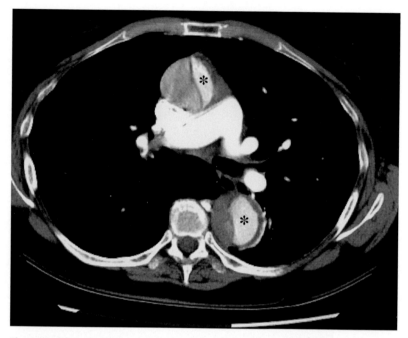

Fig. 4.32 Aortic dissection, contrast-enhanced CT. Contrast is seen in the true lumen (asterisks), whilst the false lumen is not enhancing.

Further imaging: indicated if diagnosis clinically suspected and CXR anything but normal. Local policies may vary.

■ *Contrast-enhanced CT of thorax*: through the aortic arch. Demonstrates the dissection flap and differential opacification of the true and false lumens.
■ *Angiography*: same findings as on CT, but also allows demonstration of renal and visceral artery involvement and the presence or absence of aortic regurgitation.
■ *MRI*: same findings as angiography but noninvasive. However, it is difficult to perform as an emergency procedure on a very sick patient.

Pulmonary embolism

See p. 46.

Pneumothorax

See p. 48.

Chest infection

May cause pain if pleuritic involvement. See p. 63.

Malignancy

Chest wall invasion by tumours such as breast carcinoma and mesothelioma will cause significant pain. The tumour is usually clearly evident as a soft tissue mass at the site of symptoms.

Reflux oesophagitis

CXR is usually normal.

■ Hiatus hernia (Fig. 4.33): seen as a density behind the cardiac shadow. Often an air–fluid level is seen. NB: hiatus herniae are very common in asymptomatic patients.

Further imaging:

■ *Lateral CXR* often demonstrates hiatus hernia clearly.
■ *Barium swallow* may demonstrate abnormal motility, reflux, mucosal inflammation and secondary stricture.

Musculoskeletal pain (nonspecific)

Usually a diagnosis of exclusion. No imaging features.

COUGH/HAEMOPTYSIS

A chest X-ray should be the first imaging investigation.

Chest infection (see also p. 43)

Tuberculosis is mentioned here, but the reader should remember

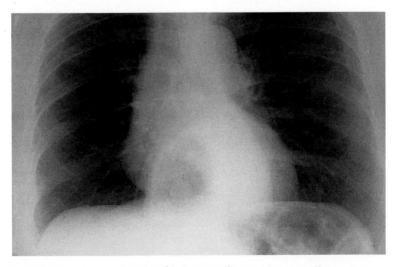

Fig. 4.33 Hiatus hernia. Typical air-filled retrocardiac opacity.

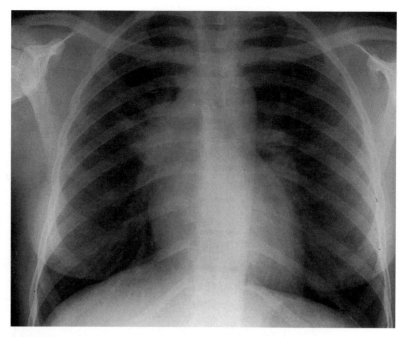

Fig. 4.34 Primary TB. There is right perihilar consolidation with hilar lymphadenopathy.

the wide spectrum of clinical disease caused by this infection, the incidence of which is rising.

Primary infection (Fig. 4.34) causes CXR appearances similar to any infection; namely localized consolidation at any site, although with a slight preference for the lower lobes. Associated hilar lymphadenopathy is common, but is not always evident on the CXR. Note that cavitation at this stage is rare, and the infection usually heals without complications. However, widespread pulmonary infection and/or blood-borne miliary spread can follow primary infection, particularly in immunocompromised patients.

Secondary infection (Fig. 4.35) occurs in later life due to reinfection. It is this stage which is associated with the classic CXR appearances of TB. Patchy consolidation in the upper lobes is seen which frequently cavitates. The apical segments of the upper or lower lobes are those usually affected. Pleural involvement with empyema formation is also seen. As with primary TB, widespread bronchial infection and miliary spread are both possible complications. Healing occurs with scarring and fibrosis, despite effective antituberculous chemotherapy. This results in the typical CXR appearance of calcified apical linear scarring, and fibrosis causing volume loss, seen as distortion of the lung architecture and elevation of the hilum. Radiological differentiation between active and healed TB may be difficult. Consolidation with air bronchograms suggests the former, but whenever possible the current film should be compared with

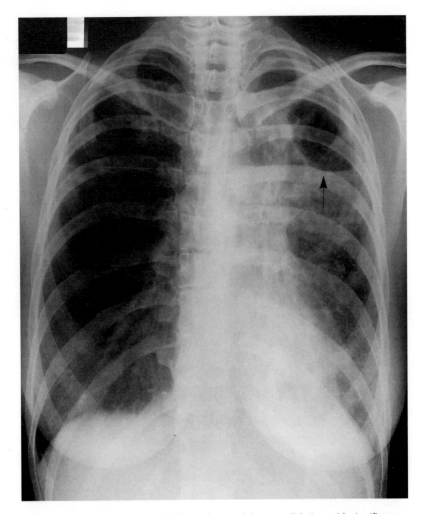

Fig. 4.35 Secondary TB. There is bilateral upper lobe consolidation with significant cavitation on the left (arrow).

previous ones to look for changing appearances suggestive of active infection.

Miliary TB (Fig. 4.36), due to blood-borne spread, may complicate both primary and secondary infection as well as primary infection outside the chest, and is more common in immunocompromised patients. The CXR shows soft tissue density nodules 1–2 mm in diameter throughout the lungs in a patient who is often very unwell. Healing occurs with calcification of the nodules.

Pulmonary embolism

See p. 46.

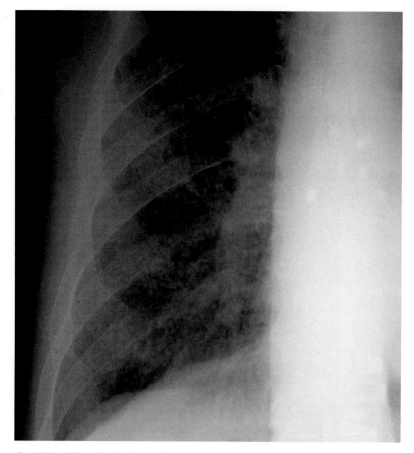

Fig. 4.36 Miliary TB. Small nodules are seen throughout the lungs.

Bronchial carcinoma

CXR features:

■ Peripheral lung mass (Fig. 4.37): there are many benign causes of a solitary lung nodule, e.g. localized infection, infarction, granuloma, benign tumours. There are no features on the CXR which can exclude malignancy, but if a lesion shows no change over two or more years it is very likely to be benign. Lesions with a smooth round outline and/or calcification are *usually* benign. Those with an irregular spiculated border are almost always malignant. Cavitation is common in squamous cell carcinoma. Note that squamous and small-cell carcinomas are frequently central tumours which may not be visible on a CXR.

■ Lymphadenopathy: enlargement of the ipsilateral hilum with a convex outer margin. (cf. pulmonary vascular enlargement).

■ Pleural effusion: exudate, often haemorrhagic.

■ Infective consolidation: due to bronchial obstruction by a proximal tumour.

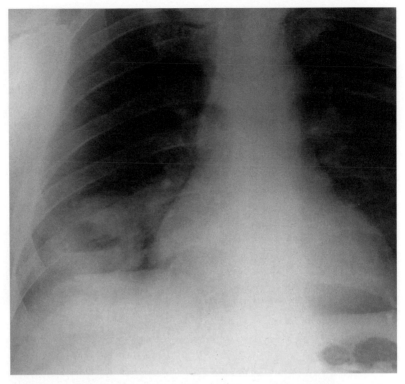

Fig. 4.37 Bronchial carcinoma. A cavitating mass is seen in the right lower lobe due to squamous carcinoma.

■ Lobar collapse: for the same reason (see p. 53).
■ Elevation of hemidiaphragm: due to phrenic nerve involvement.
■ Metastases: to other areas of lung (although this pattern is more commonly due to multiple pulmonary metastases from extrathoracic primary) and to bone.

Further imaging:

■ *Previous CXRs*: do not forget this! One of the most important investigations in the assessment of a solitary lung nodule.
■ *Lateral CXR* will confirm the intrathoracic position of the mass and allow precise demonstration of its site.
■ *CT of thorax and upper abdomen* is required for staging (Fig. 4.38). Demonstrates the size and position of the primary tumour, and the presence of lymphadenopathy and metastases to lung, liver and adrenals.

Bronchiectasis/cystic fibrosis (Fig. 4.39)

Childhood infections are the commonest cause, particularly measles and whooping cough. Bronchial obstruction due to tumour or foreign body will also result in bronchiectasis in the affected lobe or segment. Cystic fibrosis causes widespread bronchiectasis (Fig. 4.40). CXR features:

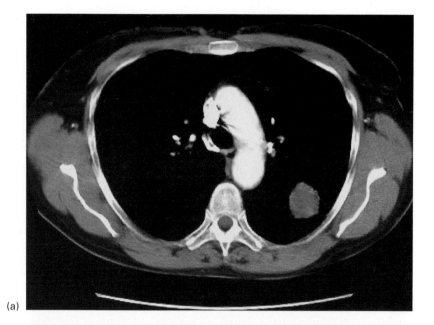

(a)

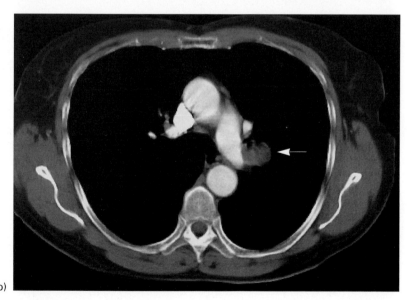

(b)

Fig. 4.38 Bronchial carcinoma. (a) Contrast-enhanced CT shows a 3 cm tumour in the left lung. (b) A few slices further down from (a) reveals left hilar nodal metastasis abutting the pulmonary artery (arrow).

- ■ Thickened dilated bronchi: the cardinal feature. Causes 'tram lines' on the CXR, usually in the lower lobes, but widespread in CF.
- ■ Localized collapse (atelectasis): due to mucus plugging.
- ■ Increased lung volumes: due to air trapping from mucus plugging.

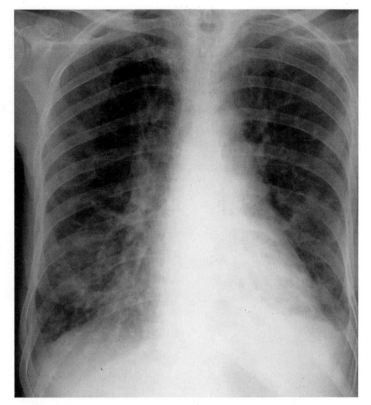

Fig. 4.39 Bronchiectasis. Thickened dilated bronchi, most marked in the right lower lobe.

■ Honeycombing: in end-stage CF. Cavities resembling honeycombs.
■ Normal CXR: in 7%.

Further Imaging:

■ *HRCT* is the method of choice for diagnosing bronchiectasis. The same plain film features are seen, but to better effect; bronchi are both dilated and thick-walled.

FINGER CLUBBING

There are several intrathoracic causes of finger clubbing, the most important being bronchial carcinoma. Chest X-ray is therefore indicated. As well as the features of bronchial neoplasia mentioned previously, evidence of other conditions associated with clubbing (e.g. congenital heart disease, infective endocarditis, fibrosing alveolitis) should be sought. Further imaging will depend on the associated clinical features and CXR findings.

HYPERTENSION

Chest X-ray to look for secondary effects, i.e. heart failure. Very

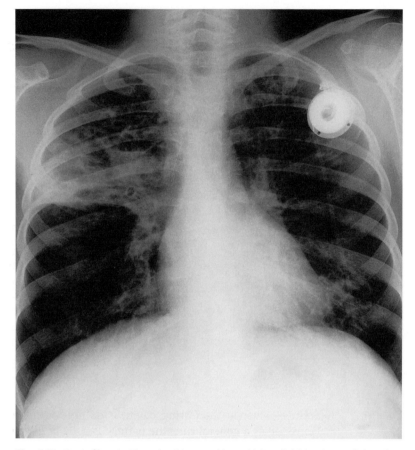

Fig. 4.40 Cystic fibrosis. There is widespread bronchial wall thickening and there is cavitating consolidation in the right upper lobe (note the long-term in-dwelling venous catheter for IV antibiotic administration).

occasionally coarctation of the aorta is seen as the underlying cause; look for dilated ascending aorta, LV enlargement, bilateral rib notching (see also p. 58).

ERYTHEMA NODOSUM

This is the commonest clinical manifestation of sarcoidosis, and it should prompt a CXR to look for associated pulmonary involvement. Even where this proves to be the case patients are frequently asymptomatic. CXR findings:

■ Normal (10%).
■ Hilar lymphadenopathy (50%): bilateral symmetrical in 95% (Fig. 4.41). Lymphoma is the main differential diagnosis; this is often asymmetrical in distribution.
■ Lymphadenopathy with pulmonary involvement (30%): pulmonary involvement has a very variable appearance; small

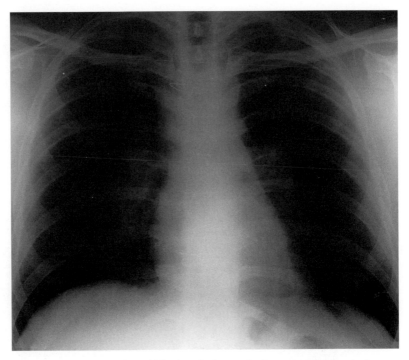

Fig. 4.41 Sarcoidosis. Bilateral hilar lymphadenopathy (note sternotomy wires).

nodules, alveolar shadowing, cavities and fibrosis are all seen. However, as a general rule, the pattern is usually *bilateral* and *widespread* (Fig. 4.42).

■ Apical fibrosis (10%): end-stage picture. Mimics TB.

Further imaging:

■ *Follow-up CXRs* to assess progression or response to steroids.
■ *HRCT* to assess pulmonary fibrosis.

COLLAPSE

Almost all of the conditions described in this chapter may be associated with collapse, and a CXR is therefore indicated.

TRAUMA

CXR should be performed in all cases of significant chest trauma. It often has to be performed AP semi-erect or supine; remember the magnification effects in such views.

Rib fractures

Often difficult to visualize, and frequently there are more fractures

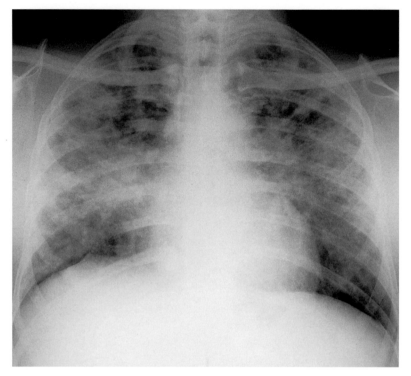

Fig. 4.42 Sarcoidosis. Extensive pulmonary infiltrates. The patient was clinically well.

than demonstrated. Fractures of the first three ribs implies significant trauma; evidence of underlying major vessel injury should be sought. A double fracture (i.e. two or more separate fractures of the same rib) is also a significant injury, resulting in a flail chest. Fractures of the lower ribs may be associated with underlying soft tissue injury, especially to liver and spleen.

Note that localized rib views are *not indicated*; management is not altered by the confirmation of uncomplicated rib fractures. The indication for CXR is to exclude associated pneumothorax.

Pneumothorax (Fig. 4.18)

May be difficult to see on supine film, since air collects anteriorly. The heart border and costophrenic angles more sharply outlined than usual. A lateral decubitus (suspected side uppermost) view will demonstrate the pneumothorax more clearly.

Pneumomediastinum (Fig. 4.43)

This may be secondary to lung tear or rupture of the trachea or oesophagus. Look for associated subcutaneous emphysema.

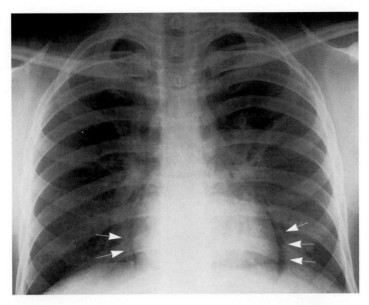

Fig. 4.43 Pneumomediastinum. There is air in the pericardium in a patient with acute asthma (arrows).

Haemothorax

This has the same CXR appearance as any pleural fluid collection. Remember in a supine patient to look for collections at the lung apices, and when seen suspect vascular injury.

Lung contusions (Fig. 4.44)

Lung opacities are seen >6 h after trauma, often at the lung bases. They resolve by 10 days. Overlying rib fractures are *not* required for significant lung contusion to occur.

Aortic rupture (Fig. 4.45)

This is associated with rapid deceleration injuries, and can occur in the absence of significant external chest trauma; immediately fatal in 80%. CXR features are unreliable, but include:

■ Widened mediastinum: but remember the magnification effects of an AP projection.
■ Tracheal and oesophageal displacement to the right: look for deviation of tracheal and NG tubes.
■ Left apical haemothorax: 'pleural cap'.
■ Associated injuries: rib fractures (especially 1–3), thoracic spine fractures, lung contusions, pneumothoraces.

If in doubt, seek radiological opinion.

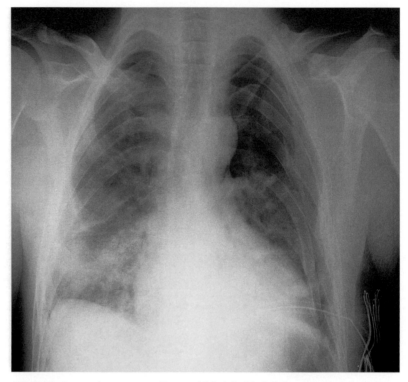

Fig. 4.44 Severe chest trauma. Note multiple left-sided rib fractures and chest drain. The shadowing in the right lower zone is due to pulmonary contusion.

Further imaging (local preference will dictate which of the following is performed):

■ *CT of thorax*: in a haemodynamically stable patient this will confirm or exclude the presence of a mediastinal haematoma. Contrast-enhanced spiral CT will often show the aortic tear.
■ *Aortography*: the aortic tear is directly visualized. When CT shows mediastinal haematoma but the site of the vascular injury remains unclear, aortography may then be indicated.

THE ITU CHEST X-RAY (Fig. 4.46)

The previously mentioned features of the AP and underinspired film and the effects of patient position on the appearance of disease (e.g. pleural effusions, pneumothoraces) apply.

The severity of illness and the frequent occurrence of complications of assisted ventilation (e.g. pneumothorax, lobar collapse, superadded infection and cardiac failure) dictate the need for daily CXRs of most ITU patients. (It is not warranted in patients who are stable or improving.)

Of particular importance in the ITU patient is the correct positioning of the various tubes and lines:

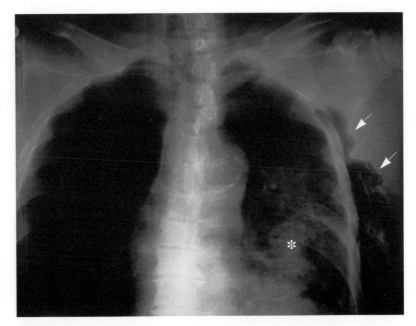

Fig. 4.45 Traumatic aortic rupture (RTA). The trachea is displaced to the right by haematoma. Widening of the mediastinum is not obvious on this AP film. Note pulmonary contusion (asterisk) and subcutaneous emphysema (arrows). Diagnosis confirmed by CT and aortography.

- ET tube: in trachea with tip at least 2 cm above the carina.
- NG tube: tip below the L hemidiaphragm, within the stomach. (Only the tip may be visible on CXR.)
- Chest drain: with all the drainage holes inside the thorax.
- Venous lines: tip in the SVC. Look for an associated pneumothorax.
- Swann–Ganz catheter: tip in the L or R main pulmonary artery.
- Cardiac pacemaker: tip of pacing wire in apex of R ventricle.

THE INCIDENTAL CHEST X-RAY FINDING

Although the 'routine pre-employment CXR' is a thing of the past, CXRs are still performed on asymptomatic individuals, for example as a pre-emigration requirement. Not infrequently, abnormalities will be discovered on these films, or on an examination performed for another reason, e.g. a trauma film showing a lung mass.

Conditions which are most likely to be encountered in this setting are lung opacities (?malignant), congenital anomalies such as small ASDs, and conditions with an insidious onset such as sarcoidosis and fibrosing alveolitis.

Clearly the further investigation and management of such patients is dependent on the possible causes of the radiological abnormality, as well as the age of the patient and the treatment options. Previous films are invaluable when they are available; it is rarely necessary to

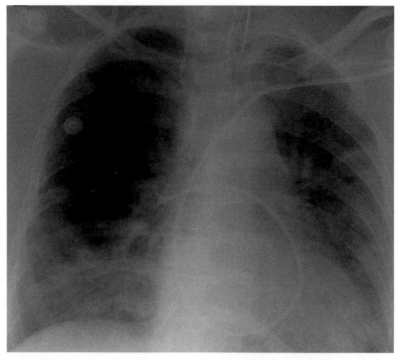

Fig. 4.46 ITU film. There are ET and NG tubes, right jugular and subclavian vein lines and a Swann–Ganz catheter with its tip in the right pulmonary artery. Note the widespread pulmonary shadowing due to pulmonary oedema.

further investigate a long-standing abnormality in an asymptomatic patient. As a general rule a wise policy to adopt is 'Treat the patient not the X-ray'.

Key points

- A departmental PA chest-X-ray is a much better film than a portable AP one. If a patient must have the latter always consider a follow-up film when his/her condition allows.
- Develop a checklist for analysing a CXR and always use it. Remember the review areas!
- Remember the significant conditions not excluded by a normal CXR; massive PE, chronic bronchitis, emphysema, bronchiectasis, pulmonary fibrosis, small central neoplasms.
- Very sick patient with normal-looking CXR; think PE or atypical chest infection (?immunocompromised patient) or disease outside the chest.
- Very sick-looking CXR with well patient; think sarcoidosis.
- With almost any CXR abnormality the most relevant (and cheapest) next test is a review of previous films.
- Follow-up films can be as helpful as more expensive, higher-dose investigations, but should not be performed too early.

The abdomen and pelvis

5

Abdominal X-ray (Fig. 5.1)

This is performed with the patient supine and the X-ray beam passing from anterior to posterior (AP). The exposure is made during arrested

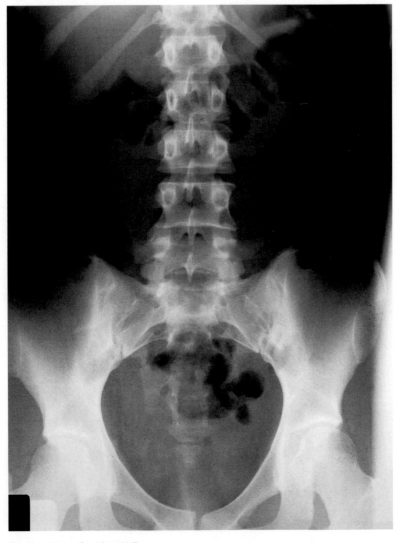

Fig. 5.1 Normal supine AXR.

respiration to prevent movement artefact. Radiation dose is equivalent to 75 CXRs. An erect abdomen X-ray is no longer performed in most departments; it rarely gives any additional information. However, in patients with an acute abdomen an erect chest X-ray is indicated to confirm or exclude pneumoperitoneum. It will also demonstrate lower lobe pneumonia, which occasionally presents with upper quadrant pain easily mistaken to be of abdominal origin.

Very small volumes (<5 ml) of free intraperitoneal air may be demonstrated by a left lateral decubitus (i.e. left side down) film.

Contrast studies

These allow the gastrointestinal tract to be imaged by coating of the mucosa with a dense contrast, usually barium solution. In a *barium swallow* the patient swallows the contrast under fluoroscopic screening, and images are obtained whilst the oesophagus is well distended. A *barium meal* (Fig. 5.2) extends the study to involve the stomach and proximal duodenum. The stomach is distended by the ingestion of effervescent granules or tablets. Although upper GI endoscopy has reduced the indications for barium studies of the upper GI tract they remain useful for assessing swallowing and motility disorders. They are also better tolerated by some patients, have fewer complications, and provide a permanent record which is less operator-dependent than endoscopy. A *small-bowel follow-*

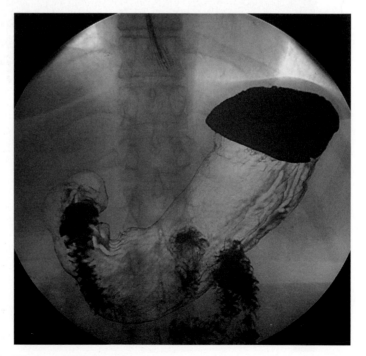

Fig. 5.2 Normal barium meal examination.

through images the small bowel by intermittent screening of ingested barium until it reaches the proximal colon. A *small-bowel enema* (Fig. 5.3) allows more rapid outlining of the small bowel by delivering a rapid column of barium via a nasogastric tube positioned at the duodeno-jejunal flexure. Radiologists preferences vary for these two techniques, which both carry a large radiation dose (approx 300 CXRs). A *barium enema* (Fig. 5.4) involves outlining the colon via a tube inserted in the rectum. The terminal ileum is also imaged if the ileocaecal valve is incompetent, which occurs in approximately 50% of patients. Radiation dose equivalent to 450 CXRs. The procedure is usually well tolerated and in most cases provides a permanent record of the entire colon, unlike colonoscopy, which may be unable to access the right hemicolon. However, the procedure is poorly tolerated and is frequently unsuccessful and upsetting for elderly infirm patients, in whom CT may be more appropriate.

Abdominal/pelvic ultrasound

This allows detailed visualization of the abdominal and pelvic viscera

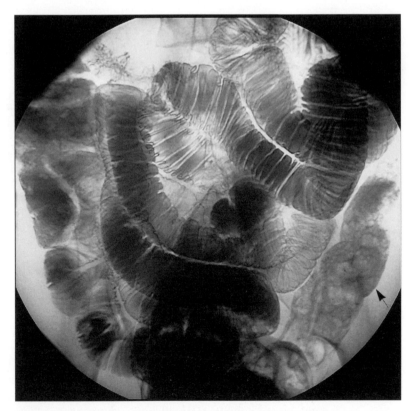

Fig. 5.3 Normal small-bowel enema. Taken near the end of the examination, with barium having reached the distal descending colon (arrow). Loops of normal small bowel are seen centrally.

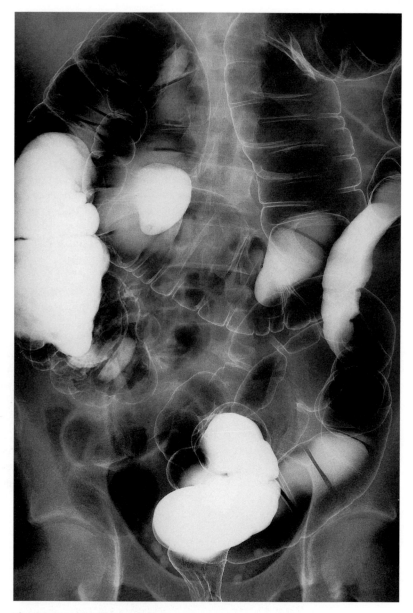

Fig. 5.4 Normal barium enema.

with no radiation penalty. Normal bowel is poorly visualized, but colonic tumours and inflammation may be evident. Ultrasound also allows percutaneous biopsy and drainage procedures to be performed accurately and very safely. The quality of an ultrasound study is very dependent on the experience of the operator and the build of the patient, scans being significantly compromised by obesity. Furthermore it is impossible to detect an abnormality which was missed at the time of scanning; the hard copy obtained provides no more than 'snapshots' of the examination. (Some departments video-tape their examinations to allow a more complete review.) In most departments, scans are performed by specially trained radiographers, although the formal report is usually made by a radiologist who reviews the images.

Abdominal/pelvic CT

This is often complementary to ultrasound and will demonstrate retroperitoneal structures and abnormalities well. It is not compromised in any way by patient obesity; indeed fat patients' CTs are easier to interpret than those of thin ones. Oral contrast is necessary to outline the bowel. Intravenous contrast highlights vessels, tumours and visceral trauma. Biopsy of pelvic masses or those close to major vessels may be safer under CT guidance than ultrasound. CT also provides a better record of the examination. The main disadvantage is the high radiation dose involved, equivalent to approximately 400 CXRs.

Abdominal/pelvic MRI

This is usually complementary to ultrasound and/or CT, rather than being the first-line investigation. It is proving particularly valuable in the staging of pelvic malignancy and in the assessment of possible tumour recurrence. Its lack of radiation is a particular advantage for young patients with haematological malignancy (e.g. lymphoma) who may require frequent scans which would incur a large radiation dose if done by CT. *Magnetic resonance cholangio-pancreatography* (MRCP) allows noninvasive demonstration of the biliary tree. Its main use currently is in patients in whom ERCP is contraindicated or unsuccessful, but its use as a screening examination is likely to increase as the technique becomes more sophisticated.

Radioisotope studies

These may be helpful in locating the source of gastrointestinal bleeding when other techniques have failed. A 'Meckel's scan' locates the ectopic gastric mucosa of a Meckel's diverticulum.

Mesenteric angiography

The arterial supply to the gastrointestinal tract is imaged by selectively catheterizing the coeliac axis, SMA and IMA in turn. This is invariably done from the femoral artery in the same way as femoral angiography. The usual indication is significant active gastrointestinal bleeding when upper endoscopy and sigmoidoscopy have failed to identify the source of bleeding (note that significant active GI bleeding is a contraindication to barium studies). Unfortunately, even in the presence of significant active GI bleeding, mesenteric angiography often fails to locate the bleeding source.

IVU

Serial X-rays are performed following the intravenous injection of iodinated contrast. The contrast is concentrated and excreted by the kidneys, which are thereby visualized on X-ray. The main indication is the investigation of renal colic and renal tract obstruction. It should not be performed in acute renal failure, and is rarely helpful

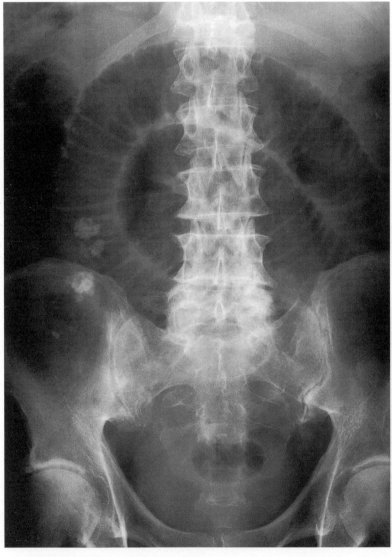

Fig. 5.5 Small-bowel obstruction. Supine AXR.

in chronic renal failure due to the poor contrast uptake by the kidneys. Radiation dose equivalent to 230 CXRs.

THE ACUTE ABDOMEN

Supine abdominal and erect chest X-rays should be performed. If the patient's condition precludes an erect CXR the radiographer will usually do a film with him/her sitting up in bed 'semierect' and will label the film as such. Look for the following.

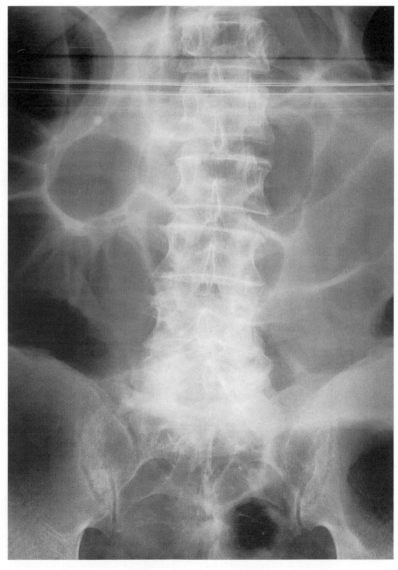

Fig. 5.6 Large-bowel obstruction: supine AXR showing widespread dilatation.

Small-bowel dilatation (Fig. 5.5)

The normal small bowel measures up to 2.5 cm in diameter and occupies a more central position within the abdomen. Look for the transverse lines ('valvulae conniventes') which traverse the full width of small bowel, helping to differentiate it from colon. Remember that a dilated bowel is not necessarily an obstructed bowel; the X-ray appearances must be correlated with the clinical findings. Localized small-bowel dilatation occurs in relation to inflammatory disease ('sentinel loop'), e.g. in the RIF in acute appendicitis; in the mid-abdomen in acute pancreatitis.

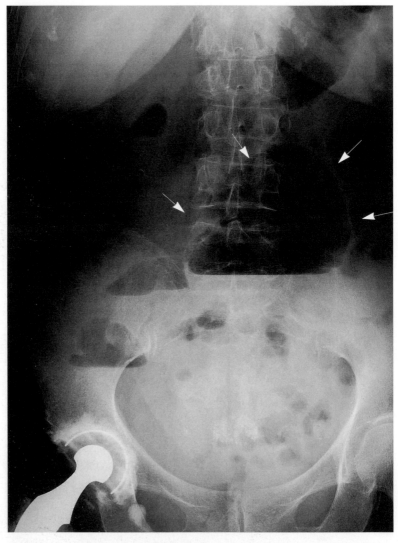

Fig. 5.7 Caecal volvulus. Erect AXR showing a centrally placed, inverted dilated caecum (arrows).

Large-bowel dilatation (Figs 5.6–5.8)

The normal large bowel is much more variable in diameter, but greater than 5.5 cm is usually abnormal. The colon lies more peripherally and has transverse lines ('haustra') which do *not* traverse its full width and are more widely spaced. As with the small bowel, a dilated colon is not always obstructed; look particularly for the caecum, which is rarely normal size in colonic obstruction. If its diameter exceeds 9 cm, then caecal perforation may be imminent, even in nonobstructed dilatation. If the ileocaecal valve is incompetent, then dilated small bowel will also be present.

Bowel wall thickening

This is often difficult to assess; compare suspicious areas with bowel loops which look normal. Thickening of the wall or haustra is seen in

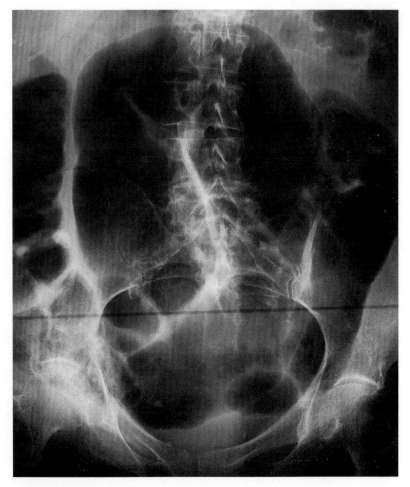

Fig. 5.8 Sigmoid volvulus.

bowel affected by inflammatory or infective colitis, ischaemia and neoplasm. 'Thumbprinting' (Fig. 5.9) is a frequent associated sign. Signs on X-ray should be correlated with the clinical picture to determine the likely underlying disease.

Pneumoperitoneum (Figs 5.10, 5.11)

Invariably due to perforated viscus, usually from peptic ulceration or perforated sigmoid diverticulum. This is a vital sign to detect. Unfortunately it is often very subtle, and is frequently missed. Free air within the peritoneum outlines the outside wall of related loops of bowel ('Wrigler's sign'). Large volumes of free air are seen centrally on the supine film ('football sign') or collect anteriorly to the liver, outlining the falciform ligament. Triangular shaped gas collections are very suggestive. An erect CXR may show obvious free air below the hemidiaphragm, but the patient's condition may not allow it; if so consider a lateral decubitus film and look for free air outlining the liver edge. Remember that pneumoperitoneum is normal following abdominal surgery. However, if a new perforation is suspected in a post-op patient, then serial films may show an increasing volume of free air. Water-soluble contrast studies can then be performed to demonstrate the site of perforation (e.g. at a surgical anastomosis) (Fig. 5.12).

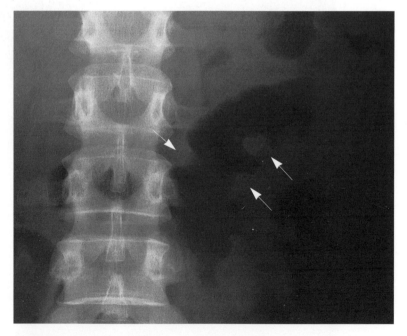

Fig. 5.9 Thumbprinting in the transverse colon (arrows). In this case due to salmonella colitis.

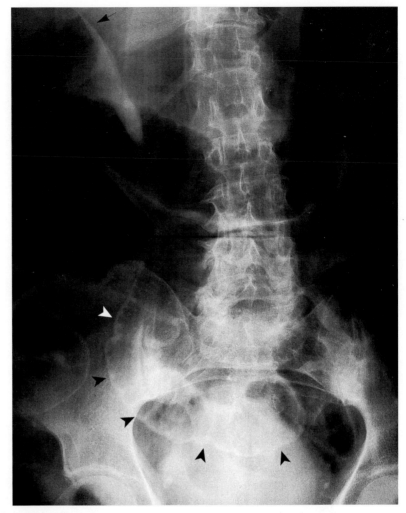

Fig. 5.10 Pneumoperitoneum, supine AXR showing free peritoneal air outlining the falciform ligament (arrow) and the outer wall of a loop of small bowel (arrowheads) – Wrigler's sign.

Renal calculus (Fig. 5.13)

Ninety percent of renal calculi are radiopaque. The line of the ureters follows the outer transverse processes of the lumbar vertebrae, then the sacroiliac joints before passing medially to join the bladder. Ureteric calculi may be very difficult to see, and in the pelvis are easily confused with vascular calcification ('phleboliths'). If the history suggests renal colic then an IVU should be performed.

Calcified abdominal aortic aneurysm (Fig. 5.14)

When seen in a patient with an acute abdomen, leaking aortic aneurysm must be considered. Unless the patient is haemodynamically

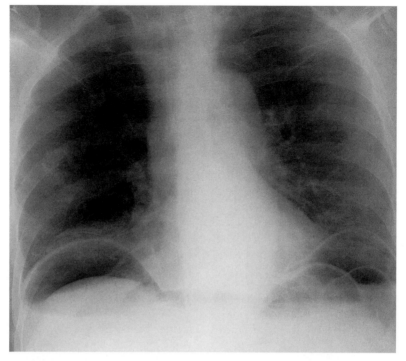

Fig. 5.11 Pneumoperitoneum. Erect chest X-ray clearly shows free intraperitoneal air beneath both hemidiaphragms.

stable, further imaging to confirm this diagnosis is *not* appropriate; the patient needs to be on the operating, not the CT scanning, table.

Causes of acute abdomen with a normal AXR

- Small-bowel dilatation can give rise to an entirely normal film if the small bowel is fluid-filled. Consider ultrasound to confirm the diagnosis.
- Perforated bowel does not always result in radiologically apparent pneumoperitoneum; a lateral decubitus film can demonstrate very small volumes of free air.
- Ischaemic and inflammatory colitis are often associated with a normal abdominal film, particularly in the acute stages.
- The same is true of renal colic and leaking abdominal aortic aneurysm, both of which rely on calcification to be evident on the X-ray.
- Acute pancreatitis and cholecystitis are usually associated with a normal film; if these are clinically suspected then an abdominal film merely excludes other causes, if it is indicated at all.
- Finally, pathology outside the abdomen must not be forgotten; lower lobe pneumonia is the classic mimicker of an acute abdomen, but acute MI, pulmonary embolism and pneumothorax can also catch the unwary!

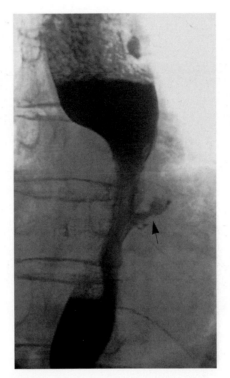

Fig. 5.12 Water-soluble contrast study showing a small leak (arrow) following balloon dilatation of a malignant oesophageal stricture.

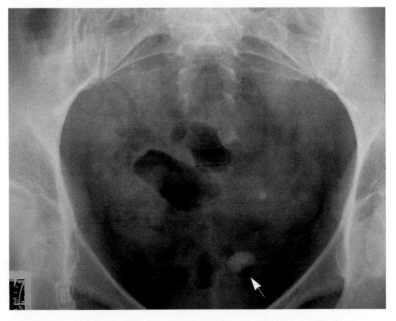

Fig. 5.13 Plain abdominal film showing a number of phleboliths and a distal ureteric calculus (within a ureterocoele, arrow).

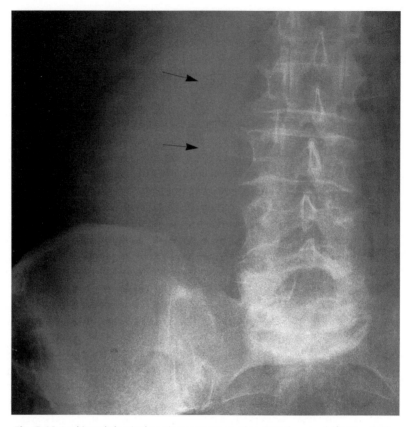

Fig. 5.14 Leaking abdominal aortic aneurysm: supine AXR shows calcification in the wall of an 8 cm diameter AAA (arrows). There is also a soft tissue mass to the right which represents retroperitoneal haematoma.

Pancreatic calcification (Fig. 5.15)

This is seen in *chronic* pancreatitis, but in a patient with an acute abdomen raises the possibility of an acute attack. Look also for a 'sentinel loop' (see above).

Faecal loading

There is wide variation in the amount of faeces seen in the colon on an AXR. However, when seen throughout most or all of the colon it is supportive of the clinical diagnosis of constipation.

GASTROINTESTINAL BLEEDING

Acute upper gastrointestinal tract bleeding

This presents with haematemesis or malaena. Plain X-rays are invariably noncontributory, and should only be requested if additional

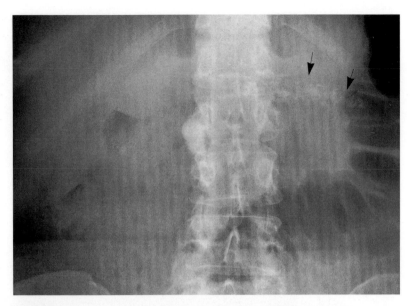

Fig. 5.15 Chronic pancreatitis. Multifocal pancreatic calcification (arrows).

complications are clinically suspected, e.g. perforation, bowel obstruction. Endoscopy is mandatory; barium studies are of no value in acute cases. If endoscopy is normal then mesenteric angiography may identify a bleeding point in the proximal small bowel, but flexible sigmoidoscopy or colonoscopy is usually performed first to exclude a colonic source. Isotope studies are an alternative to angiography depending on local preferences.

Chronic upper gastrointestinal tract bleeding

This usually presents with anaemia, with or without associated symptoms such as dyspepsia. Local policies vary but endoscopy is usually preferred over barium studies for allowing direct biopsy of suspicious lesions. However, barium studies are better tolerated and provide a permanent, less operator-dependent record.

Acute lower gastrointestinal tract bleeding

This presents with bleeding PR. When the blood loss is significant, causing hypovolaemic shock, barium studies are of no value. Sigmoidoscopy or colonoscopy should be performed first, proceeding to mesenteric angiography (Fig. 5.16) if they fail to identify the bleeding point.

Chronic or intermittent lower gastrointestinal tract bleeding

When presenting with anaemia and or bleeding PR, this may usefully

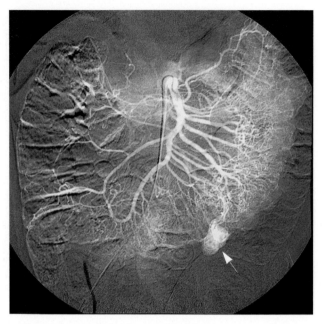

Fig. 5.16 Mesenteric angiogram. Selective SMA injection shows a contrast blush due to a small-bowel tumour (not actively bleeding).

be investigated by colonoscopy or barium enema. Colonoscopy is preferred in young patients since irradiation is then avoided. In frail elderly patients, a strong argument can be made for abdominal CT; it is much better tolerated in this group, and small mucosal lesions which CT will miss are unlikely to prove significant.

ALTERED BOWEL HABIT / WEIGHT LOSS / ANAEMIA

These symptoms, either alone or in combination, raise the suspicion of colonic carcinoma. Barium enema or colonoscopy are therefore indicated, the choice depending on local preferences. In elderly patients who tolerate these procedures poorly, CT has been shown to be effective (Fig. 5.17). Features to look for on barium enema:

- Diverticula (Fig. 5.18): out-pouchings through the colonic wall. So common as to be regarded normal, but look for complications such as strictures and fistulation.
- Intraluminal polyp (Fig. 5.19): a filling defect within the lumen, either sessile or on a stalk.
- Stricture (Fig. 5.20): irregular, shouldered narrowing, giving the typical 'apple-core' appearance of carcinoma. Strictures due to diverticular disease tend to occur in association with multiple diverticula in the sigmoid colon, and are usually longer than malignant strictures, but radiological distinction is often impossible.

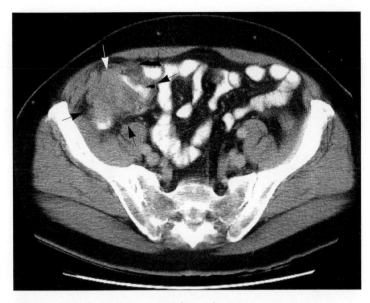

Fig. 5.17 Colonic carcinoma on CT (arrows).

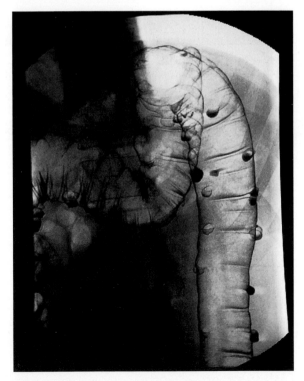

Fig. 5.18 Diverticular disease: spot view of the splenic flexure and descending colon showing numerous diverticula.

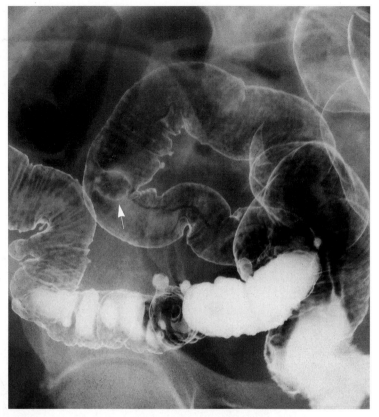

Fig. 5.19 Colonic polyp. Barium enema spot view showing a broad-based polyp in the midsigmoid colon (arrow).

- Ulceration (Fig. 5.21): defects in the mucosa of the bowel, with or without stricturing. Involvement of the rectum suggests ulcerative colitis, whilst patchy involvement of the whole colon and terminal ileum ('skip lesions') is typical of Crohn's.
- Fistulation (Fig. 5.22): usually between the sigmoid colon and bladder or vagina, or between the large and small bowel. Diverticular disease, carcinoma and Crohn's disease are by far the commonest causes, and their associated features should be looked for.

Further imaging:

- If Crohn's disease is suspected and the terminal ileum has not been visualized, then small bowel enema or follow-through should be considered (Fig. 5.23).

HAEMATURIA

Painless haematuria, either frank or on microscopy, requires exclusion

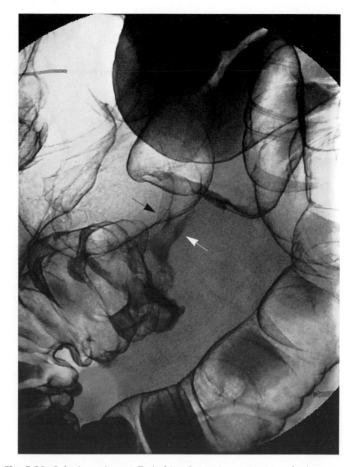

Fig. 5.20 Colonic carcinoma. Typical 'apple-core' appearance on barium enema (arrows).

of urothelial malignancy. Local practices vary, but the most common protocol for investigation is ultrasound to look at the kidneys (Fig. 5.24), plain abdominal X-ray for calculi and cystoscopy to check the bladder. IVU is performed where these are all normal and the haematuria persists. CT is used to stage renal carcinomas prior to surgery (Fig. 5.25).

RENAL COLIC

IVU is the investigation of choice, although some centres advocate spiral CT. (Ultrasound may show hydronephrosis, but a dilated system is not necessarily an obstructed one, and conversely a nondilated system may still be obstructed.) Look for:

- Calculus: on the control film (Fig. 5.13).
- Delay in contrast excretion: on the side of the symptoms.
- Dilated pelvicalyceal system and ureter (Fig. 5.26): down to the level of the calculus.

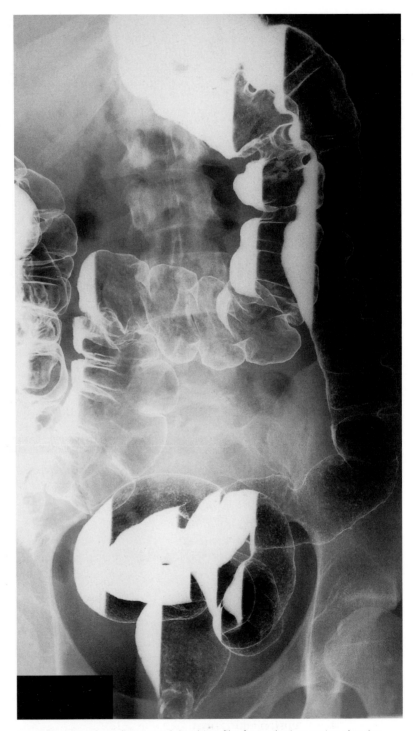

Fig. 5.21 Ulcerative colitis. Lateral decubitus film from a barium enema showing diffuse ulceration affecting the descending and sigmoid colon and rectum.

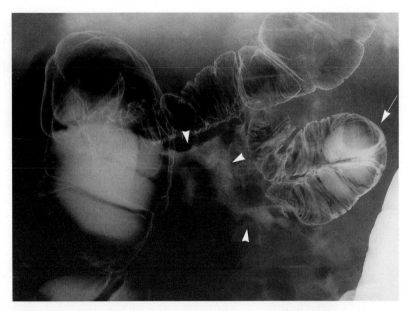

Fig. 5.22 Coloenteric fistula due to Crohn's disease: barium enema showing barium outlining a fistulous track (arrow heads) which communicate with a loop of small bowel (arrow).

Remember: colic is not always due to stone; haematuria from transitional cell tumours can induce 'clot colic'.

ACUTE RENAL FAILURE

The immediate priority is to distinguish obstructive renal failure from renal and prerenal causes. Ultrasound will demonstrate hydronephrosis suggesting obstructive uropathy (Fig. 5.27) and if appropriate percutaneous nephrostomy is performed (see Chapter 8).

JAUNDICE

Ultrasound will distinguish between obstructive jaundice, where there is usually dilatation of the bile ducts, and nonobstructive jaundice, where there is not. In obstructive cases the underlying cause is usually identified; gallstones and pancreatic head carcinoma account for the majority (Fig. 5.28).

Ultrasound is usually normal in viral or drug-induced hepatitis. Clinical jaundice due to metastases usually only occurs when the liver is almost entirely replaced by tumour. Cirrhosis is evident on ultrasound, as are its complications, such as ascites, portal hypertension and varices.

Subsequent imaging depends on the ultrasound findings. Obstructive jaundice due to gallstones is usually followed by *ERCP* and sphincterotomy. Pancreatic malignancy is usually inoperable

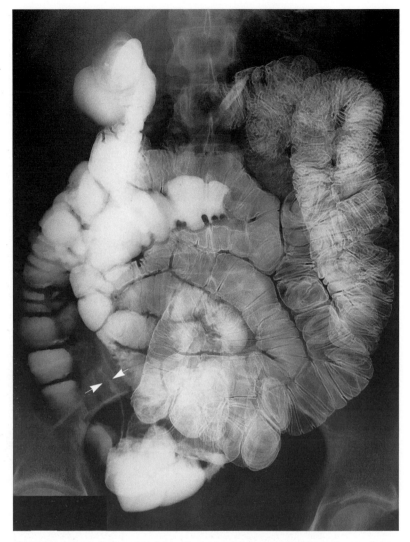

Fig. 5.23 Crohn's disease. Small-bowel enema demonstrates a tight stricture of the terminal ileum (arrows).

at presentation; *CT* helps to further assess if resection is being contemplated (Fig. 5.29). For palliation of inoperable cases, or where ERCP is unsuccessful, *PTC* allows cholangiography followed by percutaneous stenting of the site of obstruction (Fig. 5.30). MRCP (Fig. 5.31) allows noninvasive visualization of the biliary system and is likely to be increasingly utilized as a screening investigation.

BILIARY COLIC

Ultrasound will confirm the presence of gallstones, although a stone at the lower end of the CBD can be difficult to visualize. Associated

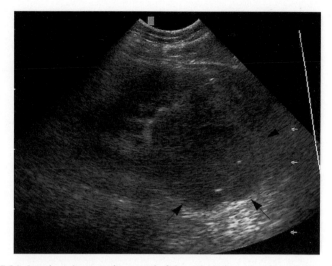

Fig. 5.24 Renal carcinoma, ultrasound of the right kidney showing a large mid and lower pole tumour (arrows).

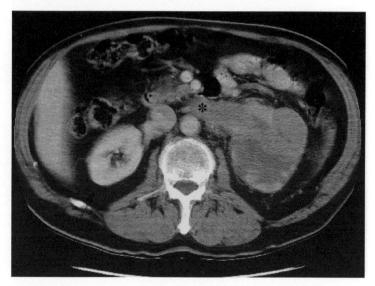

Fig. 5.25 Renal carcinoma. Contrast-enhanced CT. The tumour has invaded the left renal vein (asterisk). Compare with normal right kidney.

bile duct dilatation is readily identified. Thickening and tenderness of the gallbladder wall are reliable signs of cholecystitis (Fig. 5.32).

PANCREATITIS

This diagnosis is usually established prior to imaging, the role of which is to look for underlying cause and complications. *Ultrasound*

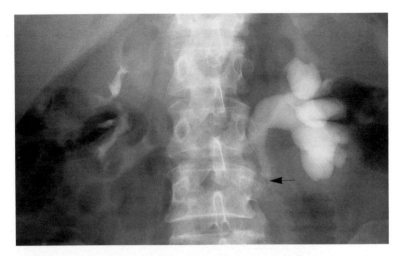

Fig. 5.26 IVU showing a left hydronephrosis due to a proximal ureteric calculus (arrow).

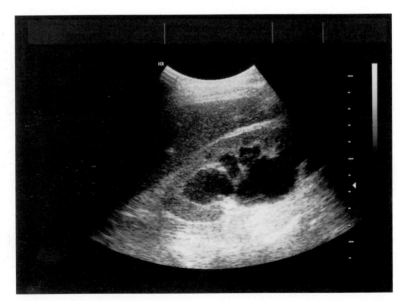

Fig. 5.27 Hydronephrosis on ultrasound.

is often difficult in the acute case; there is invariably localized small-bowel ileus which obscures the view. Nor can ultrasound assess pancreatic viability. This is best assessed by *contrast-enhanced CT* (Fig. 5.33), which allows both accurate staging of the severity of the attack and early recognition of complications.

Radiology is playing an increasing role in interventional management of these complications, such as percutaneous drainage of pseudocysts and collections under ultrasound or CT guidance.

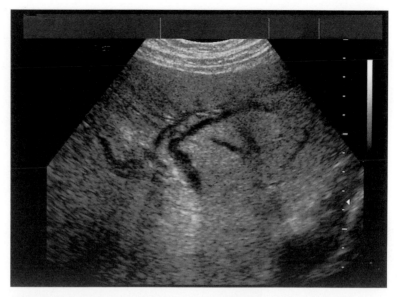

Fig. 5.28 Intrahepatic bile duct dilatation on ultrasound. In this case it is due to gallstones.

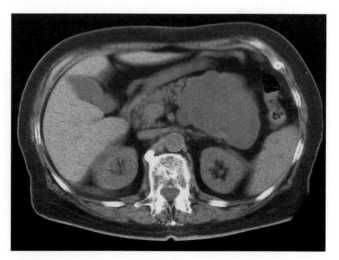

Fig. 5.29 Pancreatic tumour. CT scan showing a large low-density tumour replacing the body and tail of the pancreas. Note that the pancreatic head is not involved and there is no bile duct dilatation.

GYNAECOLOGICAL PAIN

Pelvic ultrasound is best employed in the first instance. Uterine fibroids, ovarian cysts and ovarian tumours are usually easily identified (Fig. 5.35). However, if transabdominal views are inadequate due to patient obesity or inability to tolerate a full bladder, then *transvaginal ultrasound* permits excellent views of the uterus and adnexae.

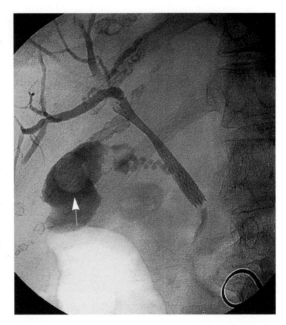

Fig. 5.30 Percutaneous insertion of a biliary stent as palliation for cholangiocarcinoma. The stent covers the common hepatic and proximal common bile ducts. Note the gallstone in the gallbladder (arrrow).

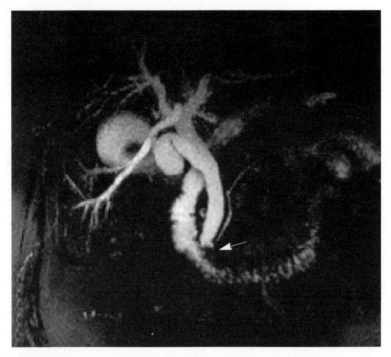

Fig. 5.31 MRCP showing obstruction due to a gallstone in the distal common bile duct (arrow).

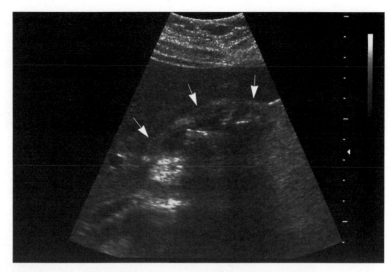

Fig. 5.32 Acute cholecystitis. Ultrasound shows a thick-walled gallbladder (arrows) containing multiple gallstones.

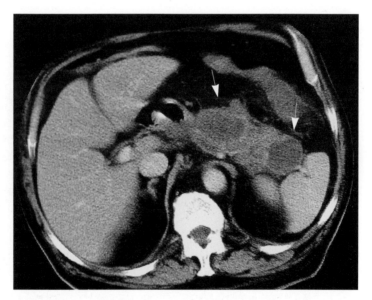

Fig. 5.33 Acute pancreatitis, contrast-enhanced CT. There are two discrete fluid collections in the body and tail of the pancreas (arrows).

PV BLEEDING

As mentioned above, *ultrasound* will demonstrate uterine fibroids. However, there is no modality which can reliably differentiate between benign and malignant endometrial disease. As such, most

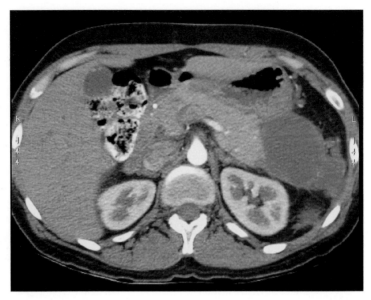

Fig. 5.34 Contrast-enhanced CT showing a large pancreatic pseudocyst arising from the tail of the pancreas.

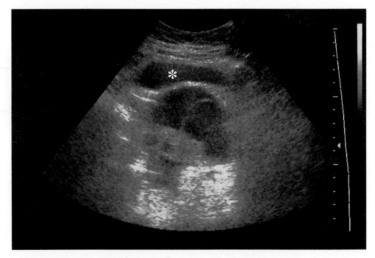

Fig. 5.35 Ovarian cyst. Ultrasound demonstrates a septated cyst arising from the ovary which lies immediately behind the bladder (asterisk).

patients will proceed to D&C without pelvic imaging. Cervical carcinoma is also a diagnosis established prior to imaging. For staging of local invasion by this tumour, *MRI* of the pelvis (Fig. 5.36) is the most accurate, although it is by no means perfect. For spread to regional lymph nodes and beyond, *CT* is just as reliable as MRI.

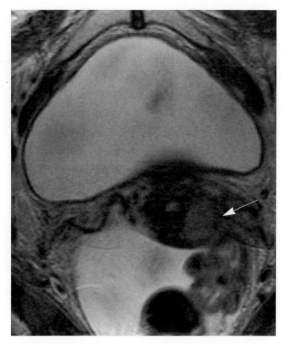

Fig. 5.36 Cervical carcinoma. MRI (axial T2-weighted) showing the tumour as a well-defined area of higher signal intensity to the rest of the cervix.

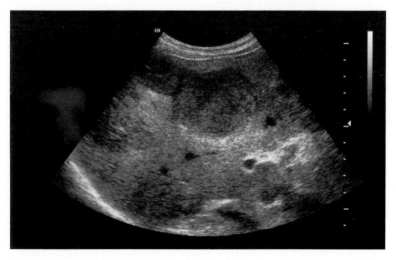

Fig. 5.37 Multiple liver metastases on ultrasound.

METASTATIC DISEASE

The finding of multiple liver metastases at ultrasound or CT is not infrequent (Figs 5.37, 5.38), and raises the important question of how

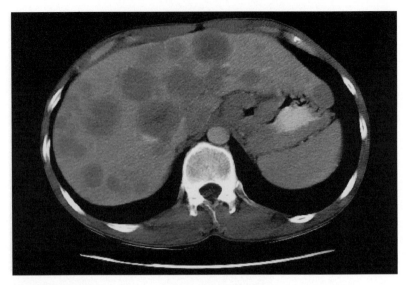

Fig. 5.38 Multiple liver metastases from oesophageal carcinoma. Contrast enhanced CT.

hard one should search for the underlying primary tumour. Careful *clinical examination* is mandatory; breast and rectal tumours are frequent causes. A *chest X-ray* is entirely reasonable, both to look for a bronchial tumour and for the presence of pulmonary metastases.

If there are features pointing towards a gastrointestinal tract primary (e.g. GI tract symptoms, anaemia) then the relevant *barium screening* test can be contemplated, although the presence of liver metastases will obviously have a bearing on the subsequent management.

In the absence of any such pointers, barium studies are usually normal, and even when positive rarely alter management or outcome. It is therefore much more useful to perform *percutaneous biopsy* of one of the metastases, usually under ultrasound guidance. The pathology may not always reveal the site of the primary tumour, but it will distinguish between carcinoma and more treatable neoplasms, such as lymphoma or carcinoid.

Radiology has a large part to play in the staging of malignancy of known origin. Well-determined protocols exist for the different primary tumours, most of them relying in some part on *CT* scanning. Newer modalities, such as *MRI* and *endoscopic ultrasound*, are likely to become important in the future. A more detailed discussion of staging protocols is beyond the scope of this text.

TRAUMA

Plain X-rays are of little value in assessing injury to the solid organs and soft tissues within the abdomen and pelvis. Pneumoperitoneum

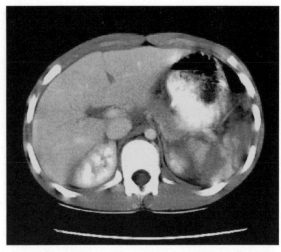

Fig. 5.39 Splenic trauma, contrast-enhanced CT. Multiple splenic lacerations are seen (compare with Fig. 5.38); this was managed conservatively without complication.

suggests perforated bowel; herniation of abdominal contents through a diaphragmatic laceration is occasionally seen. However, these signs are often absent on early films.

In a haemodynamically stable patient a normal *abdominal ultrasound* allows closely supervised conservative management. However, it is well recognized that significant lacerations and contusions to the solid organs can be invisible to ultrasound.

The most reliable investigation is *contrast-enhanced CT* (Fig. 5.39); splenic and liver lacerations are well seen, renal perfusion can be assessed and retroperitoneal haematoma, which are difficult to see on ultrasound, can be demonstrated. CT is almost mandatory when ultrasound has demonstrated free fluid. However, if the patient is haemodynamically unstable, urgent laparotomy should not be delayed to allow scanning to be performed.

Although abdominal scanning is frequently performed in conjunction with CT of the head and chest, it should be appreciated that it is not simply a case of 'doing a few extra slices at the same time as the head'; it requires oral contrast in patients who may be proceeding to theatre or who are at risk of aspirating, and it is usually time consuming because limb-splints, C-spine collars, venous lines, chest tubes etc. all interfere with scanning as well as degrading the images obtained. The large radiation dose should also be borne in mind. The decision to CT the abdomen and pelvis should be made on strong clinical grounds, and not simply because the patient is having a head scan.

Intravenous urography can be used to demonstrate renal vascular injuries following trauma. However, the inability to visualize perinephric collections (haematoma, urinoma) and the other abdominal organs means that it is inferior to CT scanning in most cases.

Key points

- Plain abdominal X-rays can demonstrate small- and large-bowel obstruction, perforation and inflammatory colitis. However, all of these conditions can occur in the setting of a normal film.
- Ultrasound can demonstrate fluid-filled dilated bowel when the plain film is normal.
- Elderly infirm patients tolerate barium enema poorly. Consider CT instead.
- Abdominal CT and barium screening studies carry a high radiation dose.
- Abdominal trauma is best assessed by contrast CT, but only in a haemodynamically stable patient.

The breast

6

IMAGING TECHNIQUES

Mammography is performed on a dedicated X-ray unit by specifically trained radiographers. Two views of each breast are usually obtained; craniocaudal and mediolateral oblique. The ability for mammograms to demonstrate cancer is much reduced in young patients with dense glandular breasts, so mammography is not performed in women under 35 years. Quality control standards are rigorous, to ensure good-quality images are produced with as low a radiation dose as possible. Mammograms are reported by dedicated breast radiologists

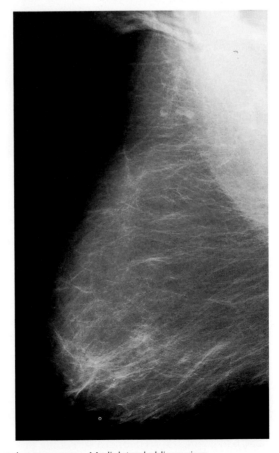

Fig. 6.1 Normal mammogram. Mediolateral oblique view.

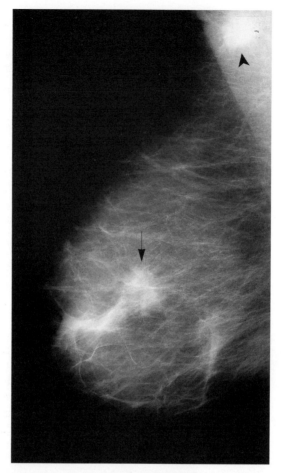

Fig. 6.2 Breast carcinoma (arrow). Note the axillary lymph node metastasis (arrowhead).

whose cancer detection rates are regularly audited in a manner unique to breast radiology.

Ultrasound helps to evaluate palpable breast lumps and impalpable mammographic abnormalities. Simple cysts can be differentiated from solid lumps, and aspiration or biopsy can be performed under ultrasound guidance.

MRI is occasionally utilized. Its main indication at present is assessing breast prostheses, breast cancer recurrence and identifying breast tumours in women with axillary node involvement but no cancer demonstrable on mammography. As in other areas, it is very sensitive, but not very specific, so the need for tissue biopsy diagnosis remains.

NATIONAL BREAST SCREENING PROGRAMME

Set up in 1988, the NHS breast screening programme is the largest of its type. Women aged between 50 and 64 years are invited to be

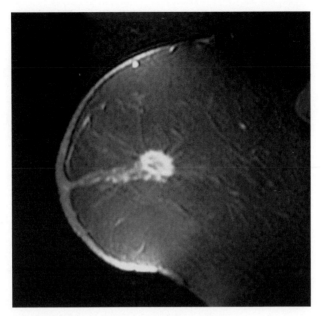

Fig. 6.3 Breast carcinoma on MRI. Same patient as Fig. 6.2.

screened at 3-yearly intervals, which equates with over one million women each year. Initially only one view, the lateral oblique, was performed, but increasingly two-view mammography is being performed, since studies have shown an increased detection rate. It is expected that the earlier detection of breast cancer in the screened population will lead to a 25% reduction in mortality, but the programme has not yet been running long enough for this to be confirmed. Trials are also being conducted to establish whether screening older women (65–69 years) is worthwhile.

BREAST LUMP

A woman with a suspicious breast lump should first and foremost be assessed by a specialist clinician, usually a dedicated breast surgeon. 'Triple assessment' entails clinical examination, imaging and histology/cytology. Palpable breast lumps are usually investigated by fine needle aspiration (FNA) without image guidance, but most patients will also have mammography and ultrasound.

When breast carcinoma is diagnosed a chest X-ray should be performed prior to surgery to exclude metastatic spread. Distant metastases are rarely present at diagnosis, so further imaging (i.e. bone scan, liver ultrasound) is not routinely indicated.

Musculoskeletal

7

IMAGING TECHNIQUES

Plain radiographs of a painful bone or joint are invariably performed, but are often unhelpful. It is important to realize that in the early stages erosive arthropathies, osteomyelitis and even bone tumours are usually radiographically occult. In addition changes of degenerative osteoarthritis are invariably present over the age of 50, and often correlate poorly with symptoms. If erosive arthropathy is suspected, an X-ray of both hands and wrists, which usually includes two views, may show the early changes.

Arthrography involves the injection of contrast into a joint which is then imaged by conventional X-rays, CT or MRI. Any joint can be imaged in this way, but it is most commonly performed to assess the shoulder and wrist.

Ultrasound is being increasingly utilized to assess musculoskeletal conditions, but is very operator-dependent. Tendon injuries such as rupture of the Achilles, and the integrity of the shoulder rotator cuff are examples of indications for ultrasound.

CT shows exquisite bone detail, and is used to assess primary bone tumours and some fractures.

The *isotope bone scan* is a very sensitive, but nonspecific way of imaging the entire skeleton. Arthritis, infection and bone tumours all show as areas of increased activity. The distribution of these 'hot-spots' and correlation with plain radiographs allows the underlying cause to be determined.

MRI has had an enormous impact on musculoskeletal imaging, allowing exquisite demonstration of cartilage, ligaments, tendons and muscles. Like isotope scanning it is very sensitive to disease. Note that prosthetic joint replacements are not usually a contraindication to MRI, but result in considerable artefact.

JOINT PAIN AND SWELLING

When restricted to a single joint a plain radiograph is indicated, but remember that a normal X-ray does not exclude significant pathology. When a number of joints are affected it is not necessary to image all areas; films of both hands and wrists are often the most useful in making the diagnosis. X-rays of the joints most severely affected may be required to determine management.

Osteoarthritis (Figs 7.1, 7.2)

Joint space narrowing, osteophytes, and sclerosis and cyst formation beneath the cartilage-bearing part of the joint are the hallmarks of degenerative osteoarthritis. Over the age of 50 years a degree of degenerative disease is almost invariable, and the radiographic appearances do not always correlate well with symptoms. However, once the hip or knee joint space is very narrowed or completely obliterated, joint replacement surgery is often contemplated.

Rheumatoid arthritis (Figs 7.3, 7.4)

Erosions are the hallmark, but are often absent at presentation when hand X-rays may be normal or show soft-tissue swelling only. It is often said that loss of bone density around an affected joint is one of the first radiographic signs, but in practice this is difficult to assess. The ulna styloid process at the wrist is one of the first sites to be affected by erosions, the metacarpo-phalyngeal (MCP) joints are the most commonly affected later. Look for a bilateral symmetrical pattern of joint erosions (just as if you were examining the hands themselves).

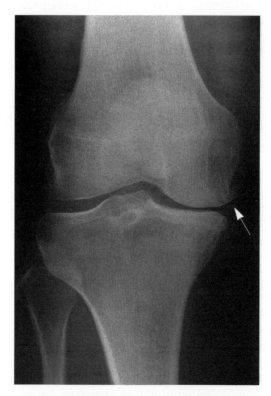

Fig. 7.1 Degenerative osteoarthritis of the knee. Moderately severe changes showing narrowing of the medial compartment joint space, subchondral sclerosis and early osteophyte formation (arrow).

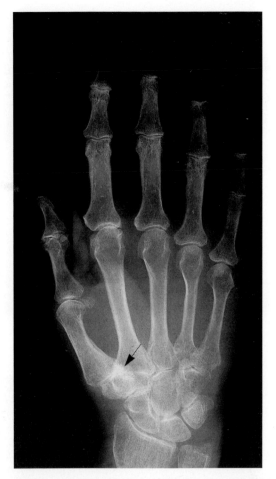

Fig. 7.2 Osteoarthritis: hand X-ray showing generalized narrowing of joint spaces and early osteophyte formation. Note that the changes are most marked at the first carpo-metacarpal joint (arrow).

As the disease progresses, joint deformity can become severe, leading ultimately to marked destruction and the classic ulnar deviation of the fingers at the MCP joints. Comparison with previous films will show the degree of progression. As isotope bone scan is occasionally helpful to demonstrate the full extent.

Seronegative arthropathies

A group of erosive arthropathies which are not associated with the presence of serum rheumatoid factor. Psoriatic arthropathy (Fig. 7.5), Reiter's disease, ankylosing spondylitis and colitis-associated arthropathy are the main ones. There is some overlap of their radiographic appearances with rheumatoid arthritis and with each other. As a general rule, psoriatic arthropathy is less symmetrical in distribution and favours the DIP joints, Reiter's disease is more

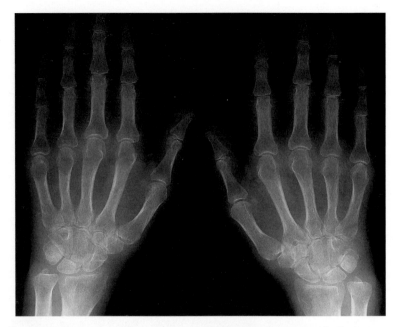

Fig. 7.3 Early changes of rheumatoid arthritis. Note small erosions at both ulna styloid processes.

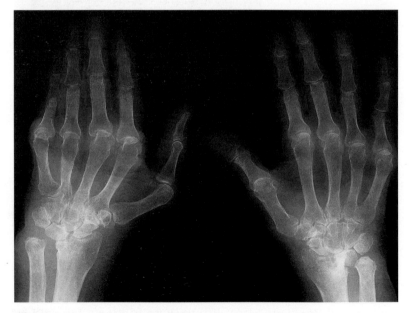

Fig. 7.4 Advanced rheumatoid arthritis. Same patient as Fig. 7.3 four years later showing progression of erosive disease at the wrists and significant MCP joint deformity.

symmetrical and usually also involves the spine and SI joints, Enteropathic arthropathy and ankylosing spondylitis affect the SI joints and often spare the peripheral joints.

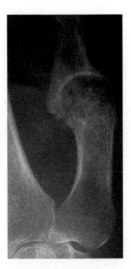

Fig. 7.5 Psoriatic arthropathy: 31-year-old man with severe erosive disease at the MCP joint of the thumb. Progressive cortical destruction at the metacarpal head will produce the 'cup and pencil' appearance. The DIP joints were also affected.

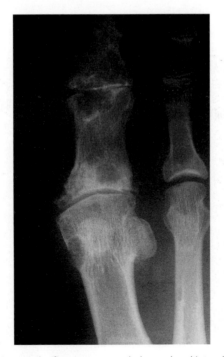

Fig. 7.6 Gout. Erosions at the first metatarso-phalangeal and interphalangeal joints.

Gout (Fig. 7.6)

The classic radiographic appearance is of punched out erosions adjacent to joints, usually the MTP joint of the great toe. Calcified tophi may be seen in the soft tissues. However, this classic appearance is now very rarely seen, since the condition is usually confirmed by the finding of a raised serum uric acid level and is treated long before such changes can occur.

Neuropathic arthropathy

The term 'Charcot joint' refers to one damaged due to loss of sensation. Formerly this was most commonly due to syphilis, but diabetes is now by far the commonest cause. The foot and ankle are the usual affected joints. X-rays show four D's; Destruction, Disorganization, Deformity, Debris. The progression of joint destruction can be very rapid (weeks–months) (Fig. 7.7). Super-added infection is common, causing localized osteoporosis and further adding to the destructive process. Confirming or excluding infection in a neuropathic joint is extremely difficult, even when bone scans and MRI are utilized. Comparison with previous films and correlation with clinical pointers to infection are what usually determine the use of antibiotic therapy.

Bone and joint infection (Figs 7.8, 7.9)

Septic arthritis is usually caused by blood-borne spread of *Staphylococcus*, resulting in a painful swollen joint which may or may not be warm. A high index of clinical suspicion is required, since radiographs are often normal at presentation. Later, there is joint space narrowing and destruction. Isotope bone scan and MRI are

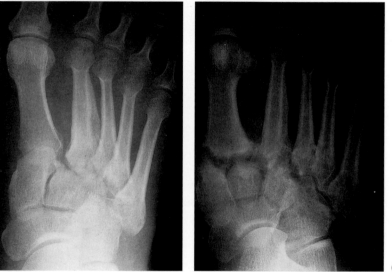

(a)　　　　　　　　　　　　　　　　　　　　　　　　　　(b)

Fig. 7.7 Diabetic neuropathy. (a) There is destruction and subluxation at the second to fifth tarso-metatarsal joint. (b) Follow-up film nine months later shows rapid progression with significant disruption of the whole of the forefoot.

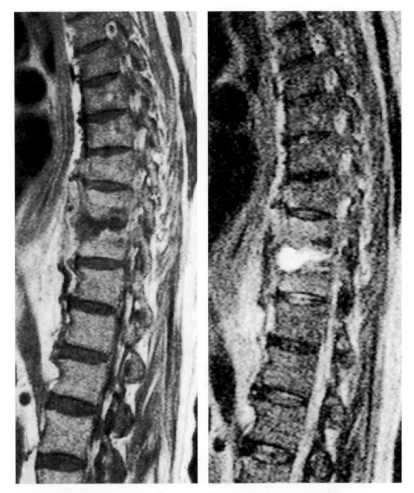

Fig. 7.8 Joint space infection on MRI. Sagittal T1 (left) and T2 (right) weighted images through the thoraco-lumbar spine showing infection of the T10/11 disc space. Note the abscess fluid collection within the disc space (white on T2) and the destruction of the adjacent T10 and T11 end plates. The plain X-ray appearances were much more subtle.

both very useful early on; they will demonstrate abnormality long before X-rays. Ultrasound can be useful to demonstrate a joint effusion, which can be aspirated to confirm the diagnosis and organism. Septic arthritis due to other organisms causes identical imaging appearances with the exception of tuberculosis, which by virtue of its more chronic course is usually associated with abnormal X-rays at presentation. *Osteomyelitis* is infection within the bone itself. This too is usually caused by blood-borne bacteria, but can also follow compound fractures and surgery. As with septic arthritis plain X-rays are invariably normal in the acute stages, but if untreated rapid bone destruction will follow. Bone scan and MRI are invaluable for detecting the infection before this occurs.

METABOLIC BONE DISEASE

Osteoporosis (Fig. 7.10)

The term 'osteopaenia' means reduced bone density on an X-ray. There are many causes of osteopaenia, but the commonest is osteoporosis; reduced quantity of normal bone. There are also many causes of osteoporosis, most of which are endocrine. In clinical practice, osteoporosis due to hypogonadism in post-menopausal women is the commonest scenario, leading to vertebral body and femoral neck fractures. On X-rays, osteopaenia is difficult to assess, since radiographic exposure factors affect the appearance of bone density. It is much more accurately assessed by dedicated *CT bone density measurement,* though this is usually reserved for younger

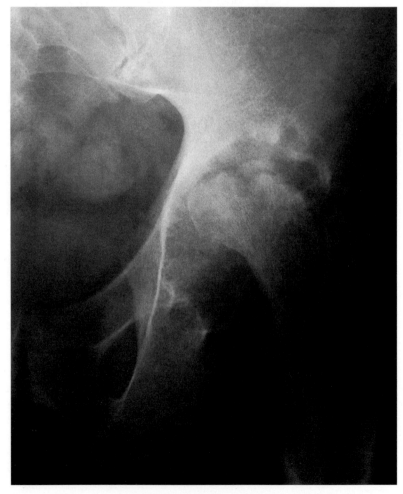

Fig. 7.9 Septic arthritis. There is destruction of both sides of the hip joint.

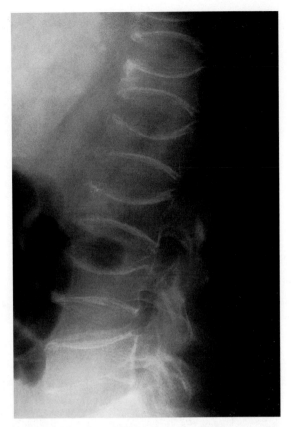

Fig. 7.10 Osteoporosis. Multiple lumbar vertebral body collapses causing the so-called codfish vertebrae.

patients at risk of osteoporosis (e.g. those on steroid therapy), since effective treatment depends on early diagnosis. Spontaneous vertebral body fractures secondary to osteoporosis are readily demonstrated on plain X-rays, causing vertebral body wedging or the biconcave appearance known as 'codfish vertebra'.

Osteomalacia/rickets (Fig. 7.11)

Vitamin D-deficient bone disease is now most commonly due to malabsorption from the gut or renal disease rather than dietary deficiency. It leads to abnormal bone mineralization, causing osteomalacia in adults, rickets in children; this is another cause of osteopaenia (but *not* osteoporosis). The X-ray appearances are therefore similar to osteoporosis, with generalized osteopaenia and vertebral body wedge fractures, but in addition there are very typical 'pseudofractures' called 'Looser's zones', usually seen in the pelvis, femoral neck, ribs and scapula. The diagnosis is confirmed by serum biochemistry.

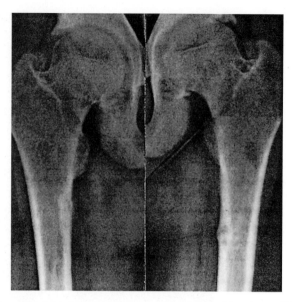

Fig. 7.11 Looser's zones. Symmetric lucencies are seen involving the medial cortex of the proximal femur bilaterally. (Courtesy of Sutton, *Textbook of Radiology and Imaging*, 6th edit., Churchill Livingstone.)

Hyperparathyroidism

Primary hyperparathyroidism is usually due to a parathyroid adenoma, with only a small percentage due to parathyroid hyperplasia or

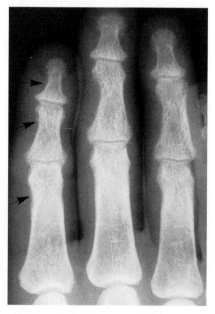

Fig. 7.12 Hyperparathyroidism. Note the fluffy ill-defined radial borders of the phalanges due to subperiosteal bone resorption typical of the condition, in this case due to chronic renal failure (arrows).

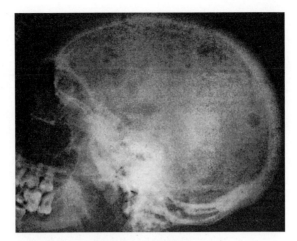

Fig. 7.13 Hyperparathyroidism. 'Salt-and-pepper' or 'pepper-pot' skull. There are multiple characteristic lucencies throughout the skull. (Courtesy of Sutton, *Textbook of Radiology and Imaging*, 6th edit., Churchill Livingstone.)

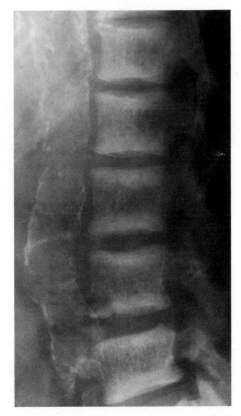

Fig. 7.14 Renal osteodystrophy. Lateral lumbar spine X-ray showing the classic 'rugger jersey spine' appearance. Note also the heavy aortic calcification.

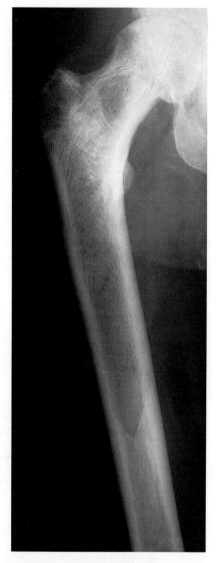

Fig. 7.15 Paget's disease, lytic phase. 'Blade of grass' appearance.

carcinoma. Occasionally ectopic production by tumours elsewhere, particularly bronchial carcinoma, causes the condition. Much commoner is the secondary hyperparathyroidism seen in chronic renal failure. Osteopaenia is again seen, but the characteristic X-ray feature is subperiosteal and cortical bone resorption, causing a very typical appearance in the phalanges and metacarpal shafts (Fig. 7.12) as well as skull vault lucencies (the 'pepper-pot skull' – Fig. 7.13). The other feature, seen particularly in primary hyperparathyroidism, is cystic bone lesions termed 'Brown tumours', particularly seen in and around the pelvis.

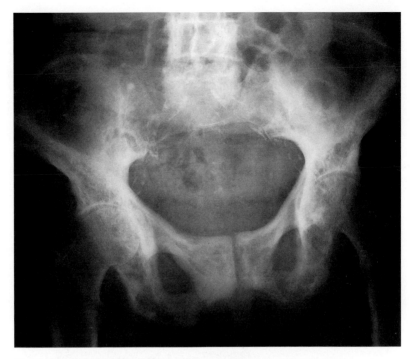

Fig. 7.16 Paget's disease, pelvis X-ray. Typical expanded sclerotic coarsely trabeculated appearance.

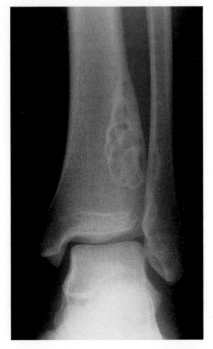

Fig. 7.17 Benign bone tumour (nonossifying fibroma). Note that the lesion is well defined and there is no cortical destruction.

Renal osteodystrophy

The bone disease seen in patients with chronic renal failure is due (as any SHO will know) to the combination of *s*clerosis, *h*yperparathyroidism and *o*steomalacia. In addition to the features of the latter two conditions described above, bony sclerosis is seen, which results in the classic 'rugger jersey spine' appearance (Fig. 7.14).

Paget's disease

In Paget's disease an abnormality of bone remodelling results in decalcification of bone, causing bowing and fractures, followed by excess new bone formation. The skull vault, tibia, femur and pelvis are the commonest sites, but any bone can be affected, in isolation or in combination with others. There are two X-ray appearances; in the 'active' phase of the disease a well-defined lytic lesion extends from one end of the bone to the other (Fig. 7.15). In the more commonly seen 'inactive' phase the bone is expanded, sclerotic and coarsely trabeculated (Fig. 7.16). It is the expansion which helps to differentiate Paget's disease from sclerotic metastases.

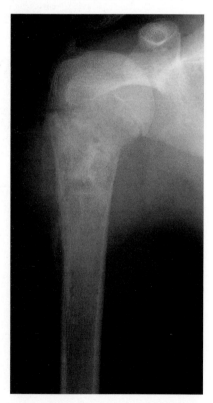

Fig. 7.18 Malignant bone tumour (osteogenic sarcoma). Note that the lesion is poorly defined and there is cortical destruction and periosteal reaction.

BONE TUMOURS

A detailed description of the many different benign and malignant *primary bone tumours* that exist is beyond the scope of this text. When a bone lesion is encountered on X-ray try to determine whether its appearances are benign or aggressive. The main feature suggesting the former is a well-defined lesion, around which it would be easy to draw a pencil line (Fig. 7.17). A poorly defined, irregular lesion which destroys the cortex of the bone is much more likely to be malignant (Fig. 7.18).

Metastases

These are by far the commonest malignant bone tumours seen, and carcinoma of the breast, bronchus and prostate are the commonest

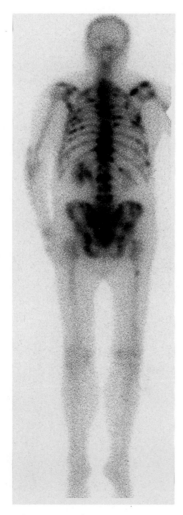

Fig. 7.19 Multiple skeletal metastases from prostatic carcinoma: isotope bone scan.

primaries responsible. In a patient over 40 years the finding of a bone lesion should prompt the search for (a) other bone lesions by isotope bone scan (Fig. 7.19), and (b) an underlying primary tumour, initially by clinical examination and chest X-ray. The appearances of skeletal metastases vary according to the underlying primary: prostatic metastases are almost always sclerotic; bronchus and breast are usually lytic or a mixture of the two. Renal carcinoma produces very characteristic lytic metastases which expand the underlying bone (Fig. 7.20).

Multiple myeloma warrants special mention; this produces lucent deposits which are often quite well defined, and which are not always seen on isotope bone scans (Fig. 7.21). In some cases, however, these deposits are not seen, the only abnormality being diffuse osteopaenia. When this condition is suspected, multiple plain X-rays of the skull, spine, pelvis and long bones (a 'skeletal survey') is performed in preference to a bone scan.

Finally, remember that bone lesions are not all due to tumour;

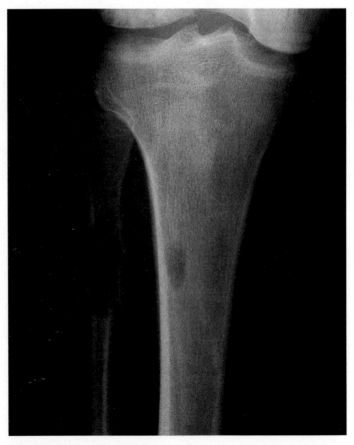

Fig. 7.20 Skeletal metastasis due to renal carcinoma. An expansile deposit is seen in the proximal fibula. A smaller deposit is present in the tibia.

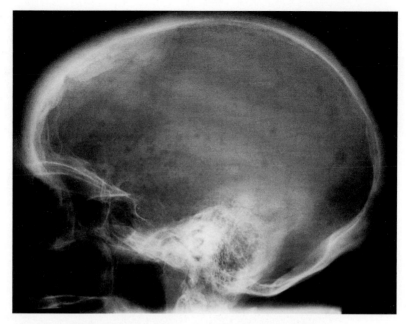

Fig. 7.21 Myeloma. Multiple small lucent skull vault deposits.

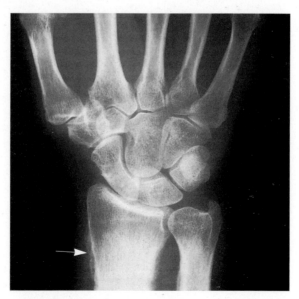

Fig. 7.22 Hypertrophic osteo-arthropathy (HOA). Note the periosteal reaction affecting the distal radius (arrow).

bone or joint infection can cause an aggressive, destructive appearance indistinguishable from tumour. Healing fractures can also mimic the appearances of a malignant bone lesion, which has even on occasion led to amputation!

Hypertrophic osteo-arthropathy (HOA)

This is a nonmetastatic manifestation of malignancy which causes bilateral symmetrical joint swelling and pain, usually affecting the wrists, MCP joints and ankles. It is usually associated with finger clubbing. There are many causes, but bronchogenic carcinoma is the commonest. X-rays show a ragged periosteal reaction along the bone shafts (Fig. 7.22), and should prompt a CXR to determine the underlying cause.

Key points

- Osteomyelitis and joint infection usually present with normal X-rays; bone scan or MRI should be considered.
- Erosive arthropathies often present with joint swelling and pain before plain films show evidence of erosions.
- A bone lesion in a patient over 40 years is most commonly a metastasis. A bone scan will demonstrate other lesions.
- Rapidly progressive joint destruction: think infection, diabetic neuropathy or both.

Vascular and interventional radiology

8

IMAGING TECHNIQUES

Doppler ultrasound (Fig. 8.1)

A totally safe noninvasive method of visualizing arteries and veins. However, it is a time-consuming and operator-dependent technique. It is the first-choice test for imaging lower limb veins (?DVT), carotid arteries (following TIA) and as a screening tool for assessing and following up patients with peripheral vascular disease.

Venography (Fig. 8.2)

Contrast is injected into the vein whilst X-rays are performed. It remains the 'gold standard' for assessing calf veins (?DVT), but in most centres has been replaced by Doppler ultrasound in the initial assessment of a swollen calf, to avoid both the radiation and contrast injection of venography.

Angiography (Fig. 8.3)

Conventional angiography involves the positioning of a fine-calibre catheter within the vessel of interest, usually the aorta. This is invariably done under local anaesthetic. Contrast medium is then

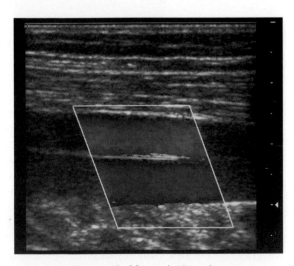

Fig. 8.1 Normal Doppler ultrasound of femoral vein and artery.

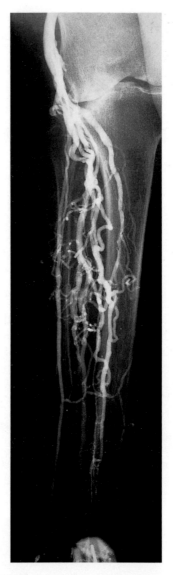

Fig. 8.2 Normal venogram.

injected whilst X-rays are obtained. The femoral artery is the preferred puncture site for most angiograms; when occluded, the upper limb arteries (axillary, brachial or radial) can be used. Diagnostic angiography is a safe technique which can be performed as a day-case procedure. Bruising at the puncture site is by far the commonest complication, and is rarely significant. In *selective angiography* a catheter is positioned in a branch artery, such as the mesenteric, renal or carotid arteries, to obtain detailed pictures of the specific vessel. This carries a slightly higher risk because catheterizing the vessel origin can cause damage, leading to occlusion or distal embolization.

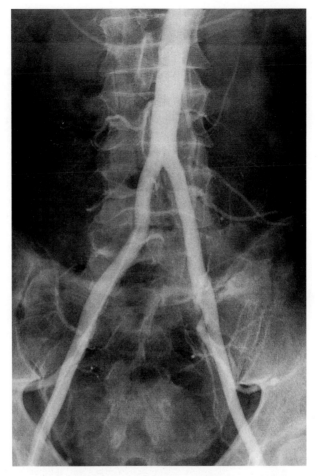

Fig. 8.3 Normal femoral arteriogram. Contrast injected through a pigtail catheter inserted via the right femoral artery reveals normal aortoiliac vessels.

CT angiography

New 'spiral' CT scanners can produce detailed images of arteries following intravenous injection of contrast. This is most commonly used to image abdominal aortic aneurysms; 3D reconstructions give the surgeon a clear representation of the morphology of an aneurysm prior to surgical repair.

MR angiography

Currently its main use is for imaging the renal and cerebral arteries, but as MRI becomes more widely available and as MR techniques improve, it will undoubtedly replace conventional angiography in other areas, e.g. peripheral vascular disease. Techniques vary, but MR angiograms can be performed with or without an intravenous injection of an MR contrast agent. The usual contraindications apply.

Angioplasty/stenting

Areas of arterial narrowing (stenoses) or occlusion can be treated by inflating a balloon mounted on a catheter within the stenosis for a minute or so (Fig. 8.4). The renal, iliac and femoral arteries are the most common to be treated by this technique, although it can be performed in any accessible vessel. The risks are significantly higher than angiography, since inflating the balloon can lead to dissection and occlusion of the artery, distal embolization or vessel rupture. However, when successful it avoids the need for invasive surgery under a general anaesthetic.

Metallic meshwork stents are used to treat occluded arteries or stenoses which do not respond to angioplasty (Fig. 8.5). They are usually deployed using an angioplasty balloon under local anaesthetic. They are expensive (approx £600 each) and are difficult to treat if they occlude, but in selected cases are very effective.

Thrombolysis

This involves direct infusion through a catheter of a clot-dissolving agent (usually streptokinase, urokinase or t-PA) into a vessel occluded by thrombus. It is most commonly performed in the setting of an

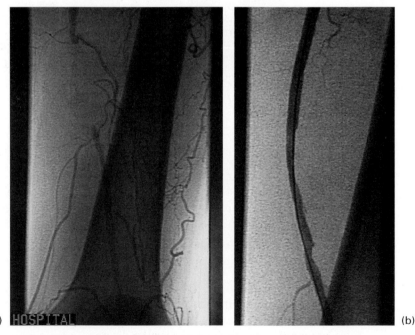

(a)   (b)

Fig. 8.4 Angioplasty (pre- and post-). (a) Femoral angiogram showing a distal superficial femoral artery occlusion. (b) Post-angioplasty angiogram showing recanalization of the occlusion.

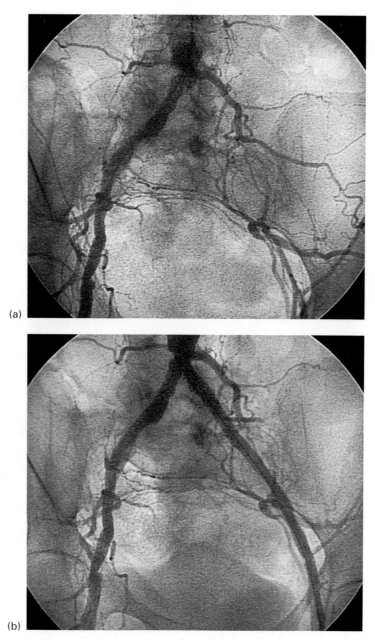

(a)

(b)

Fig. 8.5 Vascular stent (pre- and post-). (a) Femoral angiogram showing occluded left common iliac and external iliac arteries. (b) Post-procedural angiogram following deployment of endovascular stent.

acutely ischaemic limb. The infusion usually runs for 12–24 h, during which time the patient is closely monitored on an intensive care or high dependency unit. The risks are not inconsiderable, particularly in the elderly; the overall death and complication rate is around 25%, which includes an 8–10% risk of major internal haemorrhage, a

2–3% risk of haemorrhagic stroke and a mortality rate of 3–4%. However, it can lead to limb-saving reperfusion of an acutely ischaemic leg.

CALF SWELLING/DVT

Swollen calves place a heavy demand on medical teams and X-ray departments across the country. Unfortunately it is well established that clinically differentiating DVT from ruptured Baker's cyst from cellulitis is fraught with difficulty. Investigation of the swollen calf and management of proven DVT varies from centre to centre. In many centres isolated calf DVT is not treated, because the risks of anti-coagulation outweigh the risks of calf DVT propagating and causing PE. In these centres Doppler ultrasound of the femoral and popliteal veins only is performed. In centres where isolated calf DVT *is* treated the calf veins can be imaged by Doppler ultrasound (time consuming) or venography (contrast injection, radiation). An alternative to this is to scan the proximal veins only and, if negative, arrange a rescan if the calf swelling persists or worsens. A simple and very sensitive screening test available in some centres is the D-Dimer assay; elevated levels are seen in the presence of thrombosis. The test is non-specific, since other conditions will elevate the plasma D-Dimer level, but the finding of a low level can be used to exclude venous thromboembolism without further investigation.

CLAUDICATION

This is typically a cramping pain in the calves, thighs or buttocks, brought on by walking and relieved by rest. It is due to peripheral vascular disease, but only a small percentage (approximately 1% per year) of patients with claudication will go on to develop rest pain and gangrene requiring urgent reconstructive surgery or amputation. Hence imaging and treatment of claudication should only be performed to alleviate the lifestyle-limiting effects of the symptoms, and these will vary between patients. Patients must understand angiography and angioplasty carry small but definite risks, with the worst-case scenario being limb-loss. Only patients who accept these risks should be referred for investigation.

Doppler ultrasound is often performed initially, since it is noninvasive and identifies patients with disease suitable for angioplasty treatment.

Angiography followed by *angioplasty* or *vascular stent insertion* may follow. Patients who are unsuitable for or do not benefit from angioplasty may go on to have reconstructive surgery.

ACUTE LIMB ISCHAEMIA

The typical presentation is with an acutely painful, paraesthetic white limb which on examination is cool and pulseless. Urgent arteriography is indicated to determine the level and nature of the occlusion (i.e. embolus or thrombosis). Further management is dependent on the findings at arteriography and whether there is reversible or irreversible tissue necrosis. In suitable cases thrombolysis can be limb-saving, but because it takes several hours to work it is not suitable for cases with established tissue necrosis. It is often combined with angioplasty of any underlying arterial disease.

TRANSIENT ISCHAEMIC ATTACKS (TIAS)

TIAs may be due to atheromatous disease at the common carotid artery bifurcation, either stenosis or atheromatous plaque. Large studies have shown that once there is a stenosis of the internal carotid artery measuring greater than 70% in a patient who is having TIAs the risks of carotid endarterectomy surgery are outweighed by the risks of the untreated patient having an irreversible stroke. Patients with TIAs should therefore have their carotid artery bifurcations imaged to identify those suitable for surgery. This is most commonly done by Doppler ultrasound, but conventional or MR angiography are also used.

ABDOMINAL AORTIC ANEURYSM

This is often discovered incidentally during abdominal ultrasound. Surgery is considered once the aneurysm diameter exceeds 5 cm, since the risk of spontaneous rupture is significant. Pre-operative imaging helps with planning the surgical approach and is best performed by spiral CT, which allows coronal, sagittal and 3D reformatting (Fig. 8.6).

Spontaneous rupture of an abdominal aortic aneurysm (AAA) is a condition which requires surgery, not imaging. If a patient who is known to have an AAA presents with the typical features then surgery should not be delayed to enable a CT to be performed. If there is uncertainty about the presence of an AAA ultrasound can resolve the uncertainty, but should only be contemplated in a haemodynamically stable patient; i.e. when the finding of a normal abdominal aorta might avoid laparotomy. Note that ultrasound can rarely confirm or exclude *rupture* of an AAA.

VASCULAR TRAUMA

Rupture of the thoracic aortic arch may follow severe deceleration injuries, and is discussed in Chapter 4. Direct trauma to other vessels does not usually require imaging.

BIOPSY AND DRAINAGE

The interventional work performed by radiologists has increased enormously over the last few years; a large proportion of biopsies and

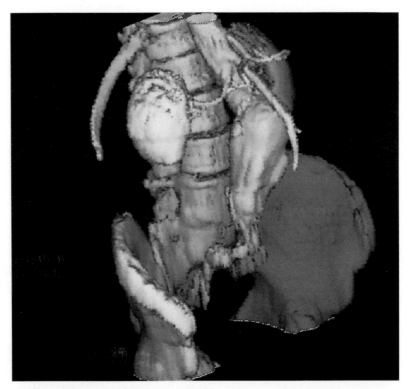

Fig. 8.6 Abdominal aortic aneurysm, 3D CT.

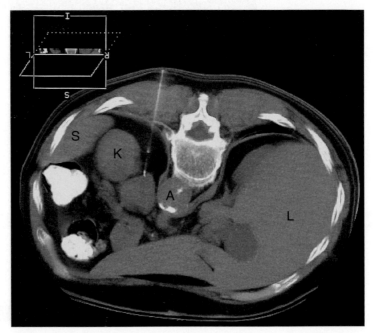

Fig. 8.7 CT-guided biopsy. Left adrenal tumour, metastatic bronchial carcinoma (patient prone). K, left kidney; S, spleen; L, liver; A, aorta.

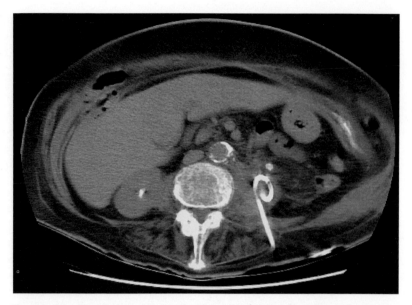

Fig. 8.8 CT-guided drainage. A pigtail catheter has been inserted into a left psoas abscess.

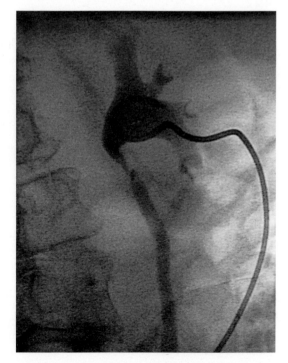

Fig. 8.9 Nephrostomy. A pigtail catheter is positioned in the renal pelvis, which has been outlined with contrast.

drainage procedures are now performed in the X-ray department under ultrasound, CT or fluoroscopic guidance. These cases should only be booked after full discussion of the case with the radiologist who will be doing the procedure.

Percutaneous biopsy

This is readily and safely performed using ultrasound or CT to accurately guide the biopsy needle into position. This usually involves biopsy of a lesion found on previous imaging studies, such as a lung tumour inaccessible to bronchoscopy or a liver, adrenal or nodal tumour. The biopsy is usually performed under local anaesthesia using an 18-Gauge 'tru-cut' device (Fig. 8.7). Haemorrhage at the biopsy site is the main complication, and in the lung pneumothorax and haemoptysis can be provoked, but are usually self-limiting. Informed consent and a check of FBC and coagulation are required. Time constraints and the need for informed consent mean that these procedures are best performed as a planned overnight hospital stay, rather than at the same time as the initial diagnostic scan.

Percutaneous drainage

Small pleural effusions and ascitic fluid collections can be easily aspirated for diagnostic purposes under ultrasound guidance. Larger or infected collections requiring more complete drainage can be treated using ultrasound or CT to guide the placement of a suitable drainage catheter (Fig. 8.8). A nephrostomy, to drain a hydronephrotic obstructed kidney, is usually performed using a combination of ultrasound to puncture the pelvicalyceal system, followed by the injection of contrast under fluoroscopic screening to allow the accurate positioning of the drainage catheter (Fig. 8.9).

Key points

- If available, a normal plasma D-Dimer level excludes DVT and PE. An elevated level requires further investigation by Doppler ultrasound. Lower limb venography is only indicated if there is an intention to treat isolated calf DVT.
- The decision to perform angiography presupposes an intention to treat any treatable lesion found (either by operation or angioplasty).
- Any patient being considered for angioplasty must understand that the risks of this procedure are small, but not insignificant, and include limb-loss. Remember that the majority of claudicants will *not* progress to rest pain, gangrene and limb-loss.
- Most tumours are amenable to percutaneous biopsy under ultrasound or CT guidance.

Index

Page numbers in italics refer to illustrations